TABLE OF CONTENTS

Nourishing Our Roots
A Journey to Healthier Eating for the Black Community

Cover design by Deborah Neal

ISBN 979-8-218-29016-0 (Paperback)

First Edition 08 24 2023
Printed in United States

For permission requests, please contact the author at dnealebook@gmail.com

In the interest of this literary work the terms "Black" and "African American" will be used interchangeably to refer to individuals of African descent. Both terms are commonly employed to describe characters, settings, or themes that explore the experiences, identities, and cultural backgrounds of people of African heritage. While "Black" is a broader term that encompasses individuals from various parts of the African diaspora, "African American" specifically refers to individuals with ancestral ties to the United States. It is important for readers to recognize the diversity and richness within the Black community, as experiences and identities can vary based on factors such as nationality, regional heritage, or immigrant backgrounds. Ultimately, the choice between "Black" and "African American" depends on the author's intent, the specific cultural and historical context and the preference of the individuals being portrayed.

INTRODUCTION

- My Journey
- Purpose of the book
- Historical and cultural context of traditional Black diets
- The significance of nutrition in overall health

My Journey

In the spring of 2017, I embarked on a transformative health journey that would shape my lifestyle choices and overall well-being. At that time, I was struggling with various health issues, including low energy levels, digestive problems, and frequent illnesses. This journey took on even greater significance for me when I was diagnosed with breast cancer in 2012. This experience had already heightened my awareness of the importance of taking care of my health and making informed choices. Feeling determined to take control of my health, I began exploring different dietary approaches and educating myself on the impact of nutrition on overall well-being. Over the course of 2016 and 2017, I experimented with various diets, including plant-based and vegetarian options, to find the optimal approach for my health. During the summer of 2017, while researching and seeking further knowledge, I came across the eye-opening documentary "What the Health" by filmmaker Kip Andersen, available on Netflix. The documentary uncovered the secret to preventing and even reversing chronic diseases through dietary changes. It shed light on the powerful potential of a vegan lifestyle in promoting optimal health. As I learned more about the ethical and environmental implications of food choices, I gradually developed a deeper understanding of the benefits of a vegan lifestyle, particularly in relation to cancer prevention and overall well-being. Inspired by the potential health advantages and the desire to minimize the risk of recurrence, I made the conscious decision to transition to a vegan diet. By eliminating animal products from my plate, I aimed to enhance my body's ability to heal and thrive. Since adopting a vegan lifestyle, I have experienced significant improvements in my health. I have noticed increased energy levels, improved digestion, and a strengthened immune system. This positive transformation not only contributes to my personal well-being but also aligns my values with my dietary choices, allowing me to contribute to a more sustainable and compassionate world.

My breast cancer diagnosis in 2012 served as a turning point in my health journey, intensifying my commitment to making informed choices and prioritizing my well-being. It propelled me towards exploring the potential benefits of a plant-based diet, ultimately leading me to embrace a vegan lifestyle. This journey has been a profound and empowering one, reminding me of the incredible impact that our food choices can have on our health, the environment, and the well-being of all beings. By incorporating the lessons learned from my breast cancer experience and my subsequent transition to a vegan diet, I have found newfound vitality and purpose in my health journey, allowing me to embrace life with renewed optimism and gratitude.

Purpose of the book

This book explores the challenges faced by the Black community regarding their diets and health from a historical perspective. It also seeks to provide information and resources on adopting a vegan lifestyle to overcome these challenges. This book aims to inspire and empower individuals to make healthier food choices while honoring their cultural heritage by offering plant-based alternatives to traditional Black dishes.

Proper nutrition is a fundamental component of overall health and well-being. Our food provides our bodies with the required nutrients, vitamins, and minerals to support various bodily functions and maintain optimal health. Nutrition is intricately linked to our immune system, energy levels, cognitive function, and disease prevention. Adopting a well-balanced diet can reduce the risk of chronic diseases, enhance our quality of life, and promote longevity.

Historical and Cultural Context of Traditional Black Diets

Within Black communities, traditional diets hold significant historical and cultural importance. African culinary traditions and the experiences of the African diaspora have shaped these diets. Traditional Black diets are characterized by a rich tapestry of flavors, herbs, and spices that reflect the cultural heritage and diversity of Black communities. They often include staple foods such as rice, beans, greens, and meats.

However, despite their cultural significance, traditional Black diets can pose challenges to health due to their high content of saturated fats, sodium, and added sugars. These dietary patterns have been associated with an increased risk of chronic diseases, including high blood pressure, diabetes, and heart disease, which disproportionately affect Black communities. By exploring the intersection of nutrition, culture, and health, this book intends to provide a comprehensive guide that addresses the unique dietary needs and challenges the Black community faces. It aims to highlight the benefits of Veganism and offer practical strategies for incorporating plant-based alternatives into traditional Black dishes. Readers can discover new and innovative ways to improve their health and well-being through this journey while embracing and celebrating their cultural heritage.

The Significance of Nutrition in Overall Health

Proper nutrition plays a vital role in strengthening optimal health and well-being. It provides essential nutrients, vitamins, and minerals necessary for the proper functioning of our bodies. A well-balanced diet can help prevent chronic diseases, boost the immune system, and support overall vitality.

Several benefits include:

Nutrients for Growth and Development: Adequate nutrition is essential for proper growth and development, especially during childhood and adolescence. Nutrients like proteins, carbohydrates, fats, vitamins, and minerals are necessary for building and repairing tissues, supporting bone health, and facilitating neurological development.

Energy and Metabolism: Nutrition provides the body with energy through the consumption of calories. Calories from macronutrients like carbohydrates, proteins, and fats are converted into energy that fuels bodily functions, including physical activity and organ function. Proper nutrition ensures an optimal metabolic rate and efficient utilization of energy.

Disease Prevention: A well-balanced diet rich in essential nutrients can help prevent various chronic diseases. For example, consuming a diet low in saturated and trans fats, and high in fruits, vegetables, whole grains, and lean proteins can reduce the risk of heart disease, hypertension, and certain types of cancer. Adequate intake of vitamins and minerals also supports a strong immune system, reducing the susceptibility to infections and illnesses.

Weight Management: good nutrition plays a crucial role in maintaining a healthy weight. Balancing calorie intake with energy expenditure helps prevent overweight and obesity, which are associated with an increased risk of numerous health problems, including diabetes, cardiovascular disease, and joint issues. Proper nutrition focuses on portion control, nutrient density, and a varied diet to support healthy weight management.

Cognitive function: The brain requires specific nutrients for optimal function. Essential fatty acids, vitamins, minerals, and antioxidants obtained through a nutritious diet play a vital role in cognitive function, memory, concentration, and overall mental well-being. Research suggests that a healthy diet may help reduce the risk of age-related cognitive decline and neurodegenerative diseases like Alzheimer's.

Digestive Health: Nutrition significantly influences digestive health. A diet high in fiber promotes regular bowel movements, prevents constipation, and supports a healthy gastrointestinal tract. Probiotics, found in fermented foods like sauerkraut contribute to a balanced gut microbiome, improving digestion and nutrient absorption.

Mood and emotional well-being: Emerging research highlight the link between nutrition and mental health. Consuming a nutrient-rich diet, including foods with Omega-3 fatty acids, B vitamins, magnesium, and antioxidants, can positively impact mood, reduce the risk of depression, and enhance overall emotional well-being.

Longevity and quality of life: Proper nutrition throughout life supports longevity and enhances the quality of life. A well-nourished body is more resistant to diseases, recovers faster from illnesses, and maintains optimal physical and mental functions as we age. Good nutrition, combined with a healthy lifestyle, regular physical activity, and avoiding harmful habits, contributes to a longer and healthier life.

In conclusion, nutrition is of paramount importance for overall health. A balanced and varied diet, along with healthy eating habits, is crucial in providing the body with essential nutrients, maintaining a healthy weight, preventing diseases, supporting cognitive function, and promoting overall well-being.

CHAPTER ONE

Reshaping Our Palate: Unmasking the Legacy of Slavery in Pursuit of Healthier Eating

- Slavery in the United States
- Dietary Practices in Slavery
- Resourcefulness and Adaptation
- Food as Community and Resistance
- Culinary Legacy and Influence
- Comparing African and Enslaved African American Diets

In this chapter, we delve into a subject matter that can be emotionally heavy but is of utmost importance to understand within a historical context. We explore the dark era of slavery in the United States and its profound impact on the African American community. Specifically, we examine how this painful chapter in history influenced not only the social and economic aspects of African American lives but also their dietary practices. By comparing the African American diet to the traditional African diet, we gain insights into the complex forces that shaped culinary traditions, ingredients, and food culture. Through this exploration, we aim to shed light on the resilience, adaptation, and cultural transformation that emerged as African Americans navigated their journey through history, connecting the dots between the past and present, and fostering a deeper understanding of the diverse influences that shape our food heritage.

Slavery in the United States can be traced back to the early 17th century when the first enslaved Africans were brought to the English colony of

Jamestown, Virginia, in 1619. Initially, the system of slavery was not firmly established, and some Africans managed to gain their freedom and own land. However, as the demand for labor in the colonies increased, so did the institution of slavery. The emergence of large-scale plantation agriculture, particularly in the southern states, created an insatiable demand for slave labor. African men, women, and children were forcibly transported across the Atlantic in brutal conditions, enduring the horrors of the Middle Passage. Once in the United States, they were subjected to unimaginable hardships, forced labor, and inhumane treatment. The harsh conditions and limited resources of slavery profoundly influenced the dietary practices of enslaved Africans. They were often provided with meager rations consisting primarily of cheap, starchy staples like cornmeal, rice, and sweet potatoes. Meat was scarce and usually reserved for the plantation owners and overseers, leaving the enslaved population to rely heavily on plant-based foods.

Enslaved individuals developed ingenious ways to supplement their meager rations. Many resorted to foraging in their limited free time, gathering wild plants and herbs to add flavor and nutrients to their meals. They also cultivated small plots of land known as "kitchen gardens" where they could grow vegetables and herbs, helping to diversify their diet. One-pot cooking became a staple in the diet of enslaved Africans. They would use a single pot to cook a variety of ingredients, often combining scraps of meat, vegetables, and grains. This culinary tradition laid the foundation for iconic dishes like gumbo, where a diverse range of ingredients and flavors were combined to create a hearty and nourishing meal.

Despite the harsh conditions of slavery, enslaved Africans managed to preserve elements of their culinary heritage. They brought with them a rich culinary tradition, including cooking techniques, spices, and flavors from West Africa. Over time, they incorporated available ingredients from the Americas, such as okra, yams, and black-eyed peas, resulting in a unique blend of African and American influences. Food played a vital role in fostering a sense of community and resistance among the enslaved population. Gatherings such as corn shucking and barbecues provided an opportunity for enslaved individuals to come together, share stories, and exchange food. These events became a symbol of resilience and a way to preserve cultural practices and maintain a semblance of normalcy in the face of adversity. The legacy of slavery's impact on the African American diet continues to shape culinary traditions in the United States today. Many beloved dishes, such as collard greens, black-eyed peas, and fried chicken, have their roots in the ingenuity and resourcefulness of enslaved Africans. The culinary contributions of African Americans have had a lasting influence on American cuisine, demonstrating the strength and resilience of a people who turned hardship into a celebration of culture through food.

The history of slavery in the United States is a dark chapter in the nation's past. The African American diet, born out of the constraints and creativity of enslaved Africans, is a testament to the endurance and cultural heritage of a people. By understanding and acknowledging this history, we can appreciate the culinary contributions of African Americans and recognize the profound influence that the institution of slavery has had on shaping American food culture.

Comparing African diets historically in Africa to the diets of enslaved Africans in the United States reveals significant differences resulting from the conditions of slavery and the limited resources available to the enslaved population. While it is important to note that Africa is a diverse continent with varied culinary traditions, we can highlight some general differences:

- **Diversity of Foods:** Historically, African diets were characterized by a rich diversity of foods due to the continent's vast agricultural resources. Africans consumed a wide array of fruits, vegetables, grains, legumes, and animal products that varied by region and cultural practices. The availability of local ingredients allowed for a more varied and balanced diet. In contrast, the diets of enslaved Africans in the United States were often limited to what was provided by their owners. They primarily relied on staples such as cornmeal, rice, and sweet potatoes, which were cheap and readily available. Access to a diverse range of fresh ingredients was limited, resulting in a less varied and less nutritionally balanced diet.

- **Protein Sources:** African diets historically included various sources of protein, such as fish, poultry, game meat, legumes, and dairy products depending on the region. Protein-rich foods were an integral part of African cuisine and provided essential nutrients.

Enslaved Africans in the United States had limited access to quality protein sources. Meat was often scarce and reserved for the plantation owners, while enslaved individuals received small portions of leftover or inexpensive cuts. They sometimes supplemented their diet with foraging or hunting, but these opportunities were rare and often prohibited by plantation owners.

- **Culinary Techniques and Spices:** African cuisine was characterized by a wide range of culinary techniques and the use of diverse spices, herbs, and seasonings. Each region had its distinct cooking methods, which involved grilling, stewing, roasting, steaming, and fermentation. Spices such as ginger, turmeric, cloves, and peppers added depth of flavor to the dishes. Enslaved Africans in the United States had to adapt their culinary practices based on the limited resources available to them. They combined traditional African cooking techniques with local ingredients to create new dishes. However, the lack of access to a wide variety of spices and seasonings meant that their food had a simpler flavor profile compared to their African counterparts.

- **Cultural Significance:** Food held immense cultural significance in African societies. It played a central role in celebrations, rituals, and social gatherings. Meals were often communal, and food preparation was a shared responsibility among community members. In the context of slavery, the communal aspect of food was disrupted. Enslaved Africans had limited control over their diets and often ate in segregated spaces. However, they managed to maintain elements of their culinary heritage and adapted communal practices by coming together during special occasions to share food and maintain cultural connections. It's important to recognize that the diversity of African diets in both historical and contemporary contexts is vast, and the impact of slavery on

African American food culture cannot be generalized for all individuals and regions. Nonetheless, these comparisons provide a broad understanding of the differences between African diets in their original context and the diets of enslaved Africans in the United States.

CHAPTER TWO

Understanding the Impact of Diets on Health

- The Role of diet in chronic diseases prevalent in the Black community.
- High blood pressure, diabetes, and heart disease statistics.
- Link between diet and increased risk for certain health conditions.

According to research, nutrition significantly affects the onset and management of chronic diseases such as high blood pressure, diabetes, and heart disease. These conditions disproportionately affect the Black community, making examining the relationship between diet and health outcomes crucial. Black individuals have higher rates of high blood pressure, diabetes, and heart disease than other racial and ethnic groups. These disparities can be attributed, at least in part, to dietary factors, including the consumption of high levels of sodium, saturated fats, and added sugars.

Unhealthy dietary patterns, characterized by consuming processed foods, sugary beverages, and high levels of animal fats, have been associated with an increased risk of obesity, diabetes, cardiovascular diseases, and certain cancers.

Understanding these connections is crucial for improving health outcomes within the Black community.

Diet's effect on chronic illnesses common in the Black community chronic diseases, which are more common in the Black community, can be developed and managed mainly through food, as research has repeatedly demonstrated. Understanding the impact of diet on these conditions is essential for promoting better health outcomes and reducing health disparities.

- **High Blood Pressure:** It's also called hypertension, is a significant health issue in the Black community. Numerous processed and fast foods include salt, which has been linked in studies to high blood pressure.

- **Diabetes:** Black people have a higher prevalence of diabetes than other racial and ethnic groups, especially type 2 diabetes. Unhealthy eating habits, such as consuming many processed foods, refined carbohydrates, and sugary drinks, help develop insulin resistance and high blood sugar levels. Adopting a diet rich in whole foods, including fruits, vegetables, whole grains, legumes, and lean proteins, can help manage and prevent diabetes.

- **Heart Disease** including coronary artery, stroke and diseases, is a leading cause of death among Black individuals. Unhealthy dietary habits, such as excessive saturated fats, trans fats, and cholesterol, contribute to plaque growth in the arteries, leading to restricted blood flow and an increased risk of heart disease. Incorporating a plant-based diet, low in saturated and trans fats and high in fiber, can significantly reduce the risk of heart disease.

- **Obesity** rates are higher among Black individuals than among other racial and ethnic groups. Consuming calorie-dense, nutrient-poor foods and limited access to fresh and healthy options in some communities contribute to weight gain and obesity. Healthy weight management can be aided by a diet high in fruits, whole grains, vegetables, lean proteins, and controlled portions.

- **Cardiovascular Diseases**: Unhealthy dietary patterns, such as a high infusion of saturated fats, trans fats, and added sugars, contribute to the development of cardiovascular diseases. These nutritional factors lead to elevated cholesterol levels, increased blood pressure, and inflammation, all risk factors for heart disease and stroke. Incorporating a plant-based diet, low in saturated and trans fats and high in fiber, antioxidants, and heart-healthy nutrients, can significantly reduce the risk of cardiovascular diseases.

- **Thyroid Health:** Certain cultural dietary patterns commonly associated with the Black community, such as soul food or traditional African diets, may have implications for thyroid health if they are consistently high in certain ingredients or cooking methods. For example:

  - **High consumption of fried foods:** Soul food cuisine often includes fried foods like fried chicken, fried fish, or fried vegetables. Regularly consuming high amounts of fried foods, which are typically high in unhealthy fats and calories, can contribute to weight gain and potentially affect thyroid health indirectly.

  - **Sodium-rich foods:** Some traditional African and soul food dishes may be seasoned with high amounts of salt or include processed foods that are high in sodium. Excessive sodium intake can disrupt thyroid function and may increase the risk of certain thyroid disorders.

  - **Low intake of iodine-rich foods:** Iodine is an essential mineral for thyroid hormone production. If a cultural diet doesn't include sufficient iodine-rich foods, such as seafood, seaweed, or iodized salt, it could potentially impact thyroid health.

It's important to note that these potential effects are not exclusive to the Black community but can be applicable to anyone following similar dietary patterns. Additionally, the impact of these dietary choices on thyroid health can vary from person to person, depending on factors like overall diet quality, individual metabolism, genetic predispositions, and other lifestyle factors.

If you have concerns about your thyroid health or how your diet may be affecting it, it's advisable to consult with a healthcare professional or a registered dietitian who can provide personalized guidance based on your specific circumstances. They can help you make appropriate dietary adjustments that support optimal thyroid function and overall well-being

- **Asthma:** The interplay between diet, obesity, and asthma in the Black community is a complex and significant topic that warrants attention. This book aims to shed light on the intricate relationship between these three factors and their impact on the health and well-being of adults and children. Research has shown that diet plays a crucial role in the development and management of obesity and asthma, both of which disproportionately affect Black children. Cultural and socioeconomic factors often influence dietary choices, leading to the consumption of high-calorie, processed foods that contribute to obesity and exacerbate asthma symptoms.

- **Certain Cancers:** Research suggests that unhealthy diets, mainly those high in processed meats, red meats, and sugary beverages, increase the risk of certain cancers, including colorectal, breast, and prostate. On the other hand, diets rich in fruits, vegetables, whole grains, and plant-based proteins provide protective benefits against cancer development. These foods are abundant in antioxidants, phytochemicals, and fiber, which help combat oxidative stress and inflammation, and support overall health.

CHAPTER THREE

Societal and Political Impact

Black Diet, Poor Health Outcomes

- The Tuskegee Study and it's Legacy
- Black Access to Healthcare
- The Societal and Political Impact
- Health Disparities and Political Disengagement

Introduction

Numerous factors, including diet and access to healthcare, have disproportionately negatively impacted the health results of the Black community in the United States. This chapter explores the historical and contemporary aspects of these issues, shedding light on the societal and political impact on Black health

The Tuskegee Study and Its Legacy

One of the most well-known examples of unethical medical research in the United States is The Tuskegee Study of Untreated Syphilis in the Negro Male. Black men with syphilis were not treated in this 1932–1972 study, even after efficient therapies became available. The Tuskegee Study had long-lasting impacts on Black communities' faith in the medical system, causing doubt and apprehension about seeking treatment.

Black Access to Healthcare

Access to healthcare plays a crucial role in the health outcomes of individuals and communities. Unfortunately, systemic barriers have historically limited Black individuals' access to quality healthcare services. Factors such as inadequate insurance coverage, financial constraints, geographic barriers, and racial bias in healthcare settings have contributed to health disparities within the Black community.

The Societal and Political Impact

The health disparities experienced by the Black community have deep societal and political roots. Systemic racism, socioeconomic inequality, and discriminatory policies have contributed to the unequal distribution of resources and opportunities, ultimately impacting health outcomes. Reducing health disparities requires addressing these broader societal and political factors to create a more equitable healthcare system.

Health Disparities and Political Disengagement

Black communities' health outcomes not only directly impact their physical well-being but also influence their political and social awareness. The interplay between health and sociopolitical engagement is complex and multifaceted. This chapter explores the relationship between poor health outcomes and the potential barriers to political and social engagement within the Black community.

Health disparities refer to systematic differences in health outcomes between different population groups, often driven by social and economic factors. Unfortunately, Black people are disproportionately affected by health inequalities, which include a greater incidence of chronic diseases, including hypertension, diabetes, and obesity, as well as less access to high-quality treatment. These health disparities can significantly impede political and social engagement within the Black community.

One significant consequence of poor health outcomes is reduced participation in civic activities. When individuals grapple with health issues, they may have limited time, energy, or resources to devote to community organizing, attending public meetings, or engaging in grassroots movements. The effects of chronic diseases can restrict mobility, resulting in physical limitations that hinder active participation in political events.

Moreover, poor health outcomes can contribute to lower voter turnout among Black individuals. Health-related challenges, such as managing chronic conditions, accessing appropriate healthcare, or dealing with the physical and emotional toll of illness, can make it difficult for individuals to prioritize political participation. This reduced engagement in the electoral process can perpetuate the underrepresentation of Black voices in political decision-making.

In addition, poor health outcomes may lead to limited awareness of political and social issues affecting the Black community. Individuals grappling with health concerns may be preoccupied with their well-being and immediate challenges. As a result, they may need more exposure to information about policy debates, community initiatives, or social justice movements. This limited awareness can hinder the collective mobilization and activism necessary to address systemic inequities.

Addressing health disparities and promoting better health outcomes within the Black community is crucial for individual well-being and fostering active and informed sociopolitical engagement. By working towards equitable access to healthcare, comprehensive health education, and supportive community structures, we can empower individuals to overcome the barriers imposed by poor health and enhance their political and social awareness.

CHAPTER FOUR

Diet, Health Outcomes and Mental Health in the Black Community

In this chapter, we will explore the relationship between diet, mental health, and the Black community. We will examine the unique challenges faced by the Black community in terms of mental health, the impact of diet on mental well-being, and the importance of addressing these issues for overall health and wellness. Mental health disparities in the Black community represent a significant public health concern. Black individuals experience higher rates of mental health conditions such as depression, anxiety, and trauma-related disorders compared to other racial and ethnic groups. This chapter will delve into the factors contributing to these disparities and highlight the importance of understanding the intersectionality of race, culture, and mental health in the Black community.

1.1 Higher Rates of Mental Health Conditions

1.1.1   Depression:

- According to the National Survey on Drug Use and Health (NSDUH), in 2019, the prevalence of major depressive episodes among African Americans was 10.4% compared to 7.7% among Whites. (Source: SAMHSA, 2019)

1.1.2   Anxiety:

- A study published in the Journal of Anxiety Disorders found that African Americans had higher rates of anxiety disorders compared to non-Hispanic Whites. (Source: Williams et al., 2007)

1.1.3   Post-Traumatic Stress Disorder (PTSD):

- Research shows that Black individuals are disproportionately affected by trauma and have higher rates of PTSD compared to the general population. A study published in the Journal of Traumatic Stress found that 9.1% of Black adults had experienced PTSD at some point in their lives. (Source: Breslau et al., 2017)

1.1.4   Suicide Rates:

- According to the American Foundation for Suicide Prevention, suicide rates among Black individuals are lower compared to Whites. However, it is important to note that suicide rates can be underestimated due to underreporting and misclassification. (Source: American Foundation for Suicide Prevention).

It is crucial to recognize that these statistics represent general trends, and individual experiences may vary. Additionally, mental health disparities extend beyond specific diagnoses and encompass factors such as access to care, cultural beliefs, and social determinants of health.

1.2 Social and Cultural Factors:

1.2.1 Historical Trauma:

- The historical experiences of slavery, segregation, discrimination, and racism that have contributed to intergenerational trauma within the Black community.

- Historical trauma can manifest in mental health disparities and influence the community's perception and utilization of mental health resources.

- **Systemic Racism:** The impact of systemic racism on mental health outcomes in the Black community, including experiences of racial discrimination, microaggressions, and structural barriers. The cumulative effects of racism on stress levels, psychological well-being, and access to mental health care.

1.2.3 Limited Access to Mental Health Resources:

- Disparities in access to mental health care, including barriers related to financial constraints, lack of culturally competent care, shortage of mental health professionals in underserved areas, and stigma.

- Implications of limited access to mental health resources on diagnosis, treatment, and overall mental health outcomes.

1.3 Intersectionality of Race, Culture, and Mental Health:

- Importance of considering the intersectionality of race, culture, and mental health in understanding mental health disparities in the Black community.

- Cultural beliefs, norms, and experiences shape individuals' perceptions and expressions of mental health, as well as their help-seeking behaviors.

- Need for culturally competent and inclusive mental health care approaches that acknowledge and address the unique experiences and needs of the Black community

CHAPTER FIVE

The Challenges of Black Diets

- Historical factors shape Black dietary practices and impact health, influenced by slavery, colonization, and migration.
- Lack of education contributes to unhealthy food consumption in the Black community.
- Limited access to affordable and nutritious foods creates food deserts in Black communities, leading to reliance on processed and unhealthy foods.
- Living in a food desert increases the risk of obesity and chronic diseases, influenced by geographic proximity, socioeconomic factors, and food affordability.
- Efforts to address food deserts include community gardens, mobile markets, policy interventions, and collaboration among stakeholders.
- The Bristol Stool Chart helps monitor digestive health and bowel movements

Historical factors affecting traditional Black diets, such as slavery, colonization, and migration, have shaped the dietary practices of the Black community.

Additionally, lack of education and awareness have contributed to the consumption of foods that are often high in saturated fats, sodium, and added sugars, resulting in detrimental effects on health. These factors are closely tied to socioeconomic disparities and their influence on dietary choices. Specifically, limited access to affordable and nutritious foods, driven by socioeconomic factors, significantly impacts food decisions. Unfortunately, many Black communities face higher rates of food insecurity, a lack of grocery stores offering fresh produce, and an overabundance of fast-food establishments in their neighborhoods. The result is the creation of food deserts, where affordable and nutritious food options are scarce, with a disproportionate impact on many Black communities. The lack of grocery stores and farmers' markets makes obtaining fresh fruits, vegetables, and whole grains challenging, contributing to unhealthy dietary patterns. Food deserts and their influence on dietary patterns often lead to an overreliance on processed and packaged foods high in calories, unhealthy fats, and added sugars. These dietary patterns can contribute to higher rates of obesity and chronic diseases within the Black community. The historical experiences of slavery, colonization, and migration have significantly influenced the dietary practices of the Black community. During slavery, enslaved Africans were forced to adapt to the available food sources provided by slaveholders, which often included high-calorie, low-nutrient foods such as cornmeal, salted meats, and molasses. These dietary patterns were rooted in slaveholders' economic interests rather than the enslaved individuals' nutritional needs. This history has shaped the culinary traditions and food preferences that continue to be passed down through generations. Socioeconomic factors are essential in determining food choices within the Black community. Many Black individuals and families face economic challenges and limited access to resources, affecting their ability to purchase and consume nutritious foods. The higher prevalence of poverty in specific Black communities contributes to food insecurity, a condition where individuals have limited or uncertain access to adequate food. Food insecurity often leads to dietary compromises, where individuals opt for cheaper, energy-dense, and nutrient-poor foods to meet their immediate needs.

Limited access to fresh and affordable products is a significant challenge in many Black neighborhoods. These areas, known as food deserts, need more grocery stores and other new food sources. Instead, convenience stores and fast-food restaurants are often more prevalent. The lack of access to fresh fruits, vegetables, and whole grains makes it difficult for individuals in these communities to adopt and maintain a nutritious diet. As a result, dietary choices may lean toward processed and packaged foods that are shelf stable but high in unhealthy fats, sugars, and sodium.

Living in a food desert often leads to a reliance on less nutritious food options. The absence of grocery stores with fresh produce and whole foods can limit the availability of healthier choices. Instead, individuals may rely on highly processed and calorie-dense foods that are readily available and affordable in their neighborhoods. These dietary patterns contribute to higher rates of obesity, diabetes, and other diet-related chronic diseases within the Black community.

Food deserts can occur due to various factors, including:

- **Geographic proximity:** Some neighborhoods lack supermarkets, grocery stores, or farmers' markets within a reasonable distance. This can be due to limited infrastructure, zoning regulations, or a lack of market demand in low-income areas.

- **Socioeconomic factors:** Food deserts are more prevalent in economically disadvantaged communities, where residents may have lower incomes and limited transportation options. This makes it difficult to access food retailers located outside their neighborhoods.

- **Food affordability:** Even if food options are available in food deserts, the cost of fresh and nutritious food may be higher compared to processed and unhealthy options. This financial barrier can further restrict access to healthier choices.

The consequences of living in a food desert can be significant for individuals and communities. Limited access to nutritious food can lead to poor dietary choices, increased consumption of unhealthy processed foods, and a higher risk of diet-related health issues such as obesity, diabetes, and cardiovascular diseases. Additionally, food deserts can exacerbate existing health disparities and contribute to social and economic inequities.

Efforts are being made to address food deserts and improve food access in underserved communities. These include:

- **Community gardens and urban agriculture:** Initiatives that promote local food production and community gardens can provide residents with fresh produce and foster community engagement.

- **Mobile markets and food delivery programs:** Mobile markets and food delivery services bring fresh produce and groceries directly to neighborhoods lacking access to traditional food retailers.

- **Policy interventions:** Governments and organizations may implement policies and incentives to encourage the establishment of grocery stores or farmers' markets in food deserts. These can include tax breaks, grants, or zoning changes to support food access initiatives.

- **Education and nutrition programs:** Providing nutrition education, cooking classes, and resources on healthy eating can empower residents to make informed food choices and prioritize their health.

- **Nonprofit and community partnerships:** Collaborations between nonprofits, community organizations, and local businesses can help address food deserts by implementing sustainable solutions and advocating for policy changes.

It's worth noting that the term "food desert" has received some criticism for oversimplifying complex issues related to food access. Some argue that the concept fails to address the underlying systemic problems of poverty, racial disparities, and inequalities that contribute to food insecurity. Nevertheless, the term continues to be used to highlight the need for equitable access to nutritious food for all communities. One important tool for understanding digestive health is the Bristol Stool Chart:

[Bristol_Stool_Chart_PDF-compressed.pdf (continence.org.au)](#)

The Bristol Stool Chart is a visual guide that helps individuals identify and monitor the consistency and shape of their bowel movements. It consists of seven different types of stools, ranging from hard lumps (Type 1) to watery stools (Type 7). By examining your stool using this chart, you can gain valuable insights into your digestive function and overall health. Monitoring your stool regularly can help you identify potential issues such as constipation, diarrhea, or other gastrointestinal concerns. Understanding and maintaining healthy bowel movements is crucial for optimal digestion and nutrient absorption. By incorporating the Bristol Stool Chart into our journey towards healthier eating, we can develop a better understanding of our digestive health and make informed choices to nourish our bodies effectively.

Bowel movements:

The frequency of bowel movements can vary from person to person. While there is no specific "normal" frequency, a general guideline is to have regular bowel movements that are comfortable and consistent for you. For most individuals, having a bowel movement anywhere from three times per day to three times per week is considered within the range of normal. Factors that can influence bowel movement frequency include diet, hydration, physical activity, and individual differences in digestion. It's important to pay attention to any significant changes in your regular bowel habits, such as a sudden increase or decrease in frequency, as it could indicate an underlying health issue. If you have concerns about your bowel movements or notice any persistent changes, it's recommended to consult with a healthcare professional who can provide personalized advice based on your specific circumstances and medical history. They can help determine what is normal for you and address any potential concerns or imbalances in your digestive health.

5.1. Black Childhood, Obesity, and Health Outcomes

Childhood obesity is a pressing public health concern, and the Black community faces disproportionately high rates of obesity among children. The consumption of sugar, fast food and processed food plays a significant role in the development of obesity in this population. Here are some key points to consider: Black children experience higher rates of obesity compared to their peers. According to a study published in the Journal of the American Medical Association, Black children have a 40% higher prevalence of obesity compared to White children in the United States (Ogden et al., 2018). Various factors, including dietary choices, influence this disparity.

- **Sugar consumption:** Excessive sugar intake, especially from sugary beverages and processed snacks, is strongly associated with weight gain and obesity in children. Higher sugar consumption was found to be positively associated with weight increase and obesity in Black children, according to research published in the American Journal of Clinical Nutrition (Skinner et al., 2018). Children consume more sugar due to increased accessibility and marketing of sugary products in Black neighborhoods.

- **Fast food and Processed food**: The consumption of fast food and processed food is prevalent among children and is linked to an increased risk of obesity. Black children have been shown to have higher fast-food consumption than White children (Powell et al., 2007). Fast food meals and processed snacks are often high in calories, unhealthy fats, added sugars, and sodium, significantly contributing to excessive calorie intake and weight gain.

- **Limited access to healthy food options:** Black communities often face limited access to affordable, nutritious food options. This lack of access, commonly referred to as food deserts, forces many families to rely on convenience stores and fast-food restaurants as their primary sources of sustenance. The absence of grocery stores with fresh produce and healthier food choices contributes to the reliance on energy-dense, nutrient-poor options.

- **Role of Marketing and Advertising:** The marketing and advertising of unhealthy food products heavily target children, especially those from minority communities. Black children are exposed to disproportionate advertisements promoting sugary drinks, fast food, and processed snacks. These marketing tactics influence children's food preferences and contribute to the consumption of unhealthy foods.

Addressing these challenges requires a comprehensive approach involving multiple stakeholders. Policies and interventions that promote access to affordable, healthy foods in underserved communities are crucial. This includes initiatives such as community gardens, farmers' markets, and collaborations with local organizations to increase the availability of fresh produce. Nutrition education programs that are culturally sensitive and emphasize the importance of reducing sugar, fast food, and processed food consumption should be implemented in schools and community settings.

5.1.1 Fast Food and Processed Food and how it is impacting our Children from 1960 to now

The impact of processed fast food on children's health from the 1960s to the present has been a growing concern. Here are some key points regarding this topic:

- **Rise in Consumption:** Over time, there has been a considerable increase in the intake of processed fast food, which has led to children developing poor eating habits. Fast food frequently lacks vital nutrients while being heavy in calories, harmful fats, carbohydrates, and sodium.

- **Negative Health Effects**: Include obesity, type 2 diabetes, high blood pressure, and abnormally high cholesterol levels in youngsters who regularly consume processed fast food. The likelihood of formulating chronic diseases later in life is increased by certain health issues, which may have long-term effects.

- **Impact on Nutrition:** Processed fast food is typically low in nutritional value, providing little to no fresh fruits, vegetables, whole grains, or lean proteins. This can lead to nutrient deficiencies and imbalances in children's diets, affecting their overall growth and development.

- **Marketing to Children**: Fast food chains heavily market their products to Black children through advertisements, packaging, and promotional campaigns. These marketing tactics often use colorful visuals, mascots, and incentives to attract young consumers, contributing to their desire for unhealthy food choices.

- **Convenience and Affordability:** Processed fast food is often perceived as convenient and affordable, making it an appealing option for low-income families. However, the long-term health consequences outweigh the short-term convenience and the affordability aspect can be misleading when considering the potential healthcare costs associated with poor health outcomes.

- **Influence on Eating Habits:** Regularly consuming processed fast food can shape children's taste preferences and eating habits, leading to a selection of high-calorie, low-nutrient foods. This can create a cycle of unhealthy eating that is challenging to break, impacting their long-term health and well-being.

- **Role of Parents and Caregivers:** Parents and caregivers play a crucial role in shaping children's dietary choices and habits. By promoting nutritious meals and teaching children about healthy eating, parents and caregivers can help mitigate the impact of processed fast food on their children's health.

It is essential for policymakers, healthcare professionals, parents, and the food industry to work together to address the impact of processed fast food on children's health. This can involve implementing policies that promote healthier food options in schools, increasing access to affordable and nutritious foods and raising awareness about the importance of a balanced diet for children's well-being.

CHAPTER SIX

Water: The Remarkable Benefits of Staying Hydrated

Water is often referred to as the elixir of life and for good reason. Our bodies are composed of approximately 60% water, and maintaining adequate hydration levels is crucial for overall health and well-being. In this chapter, we will explore the remarkable benefits of staying hydrated and drinking plenty of water. Each benefit will be supported by scientific studies, articles, and references, highlighting the significance of hydration for optimal functioning.

Recommended Daily Water Intake:

The daily water intake recommendation varies depending on factors such as age, sex, physical activity level, and climate. A general guideline is to aim for about 8 cups (64 ounces) of water per day. However, individual needs may differ, and it's important to listen to your body's thirst cues. In certain circumstances, such as intense physical activity or hot weather, increasing water intake is crucial to compensate for fluid loss through sweat.

Benefits of Proper Hydration:

   a. Skin Health: Proper hydration plays a significant role in maintaining healthy skin. Drinking an adequate amount of water can improve skin elasticity, promote a radiant complexion, and support the natural detoxification process of the skin (Palma et al., 2015).
   b. Joint Health: Water acts as a lubricant for the joints and helps cushion them, promoting joint flexibility and reducing the risk of

joint-related discomfort (Shakoor et al., 2012).

   c. Temperature Regulation: Adequate hydration is essential for maintaining normal body temperature. Water helps regulate body heat through processes such as sweat production and evaporation (Kenefick et al., 2018).

   d. Kidney Health: Sufficient water intake supports kidney function by assisting in the filtration of waste products from the blood and promoting urine formation (Strippoli et al., 2020).

Additional Benefits of Staying Hydrated:

1. **Improved Physical Performance:**
   Hydration plays a pivotal role in athletic performance and physical exertion. Studies have consistently shown that even mild dehydration can negatively impact exercise performance (Sawka et al., 2007). Dehydration can lead to reduced endurance, increased fatigue, decreased coordination, and impaired cognitive function (Adan, Serra-Grabulosa, & Reyner, 2019). It is essential to maintain proper hydration before, during, and after physical activity to maximize performance and prevent dehydration-related complications.

2. **Enhanced Cognitive Function:**
   Water intake has a direct impact on brain function and cognitive performance. Studies have demonstrated that even mild dehydration can impair cognitive abilities such as attention, concentration, memory, and mood (Benton & Young, 2015). Proper hydration helps to optimize brain function by ensuring the efficient delivery of nutrients and oxygen, as well as the removal of metabolic waste products (Popkin et al., 2010). Maintaining adequate hydration levels throughout the day is vital for maintaining optimal cognitive performance.

3. **Weight Management and Appetite Control:**
   Drinking water can be an effective tool for weight management and appetite control. Research suggests that consuming water before meals can lead to reduced calorie intake and increased satiety (Dennis et al., 2010). Water-rich foods and beverages also

tend to have a lower energy density, meaning they provide fewer calories per gram (Stookey et al., 2012). Staying hydrated can support weight loss efforts and help maintain a healthy body weight.

4. **Improved Digestion and Detoxification:**
Adequate hydration is essential for maintaining healthy digestion and promoting regular bowel movements. Water aids in the digestion and absorption of nutrients, while also preventing constipation by keeping the stool soft and easy to pass (Eltorai, 2021). Additionally, proper hydration supports kidney function, allowing for efficient detoxification and elimination of waste products from the body (Roumeliotis et al., 2020). Drinking enough water is crucial for maintaining a healthy digestive system and promoting overall detoxification.

Tap Water vs. Bottled Water:

a. Safety and Regulations: Tap water is strictly regulated by government bodies, such as the Environmental Protection Agency (EPA) in the United States, to ensure it meets quality standards. Municipal water treatment facilities employ processes to remove contaminants and provide safe drinking water. On the other hand, bottled water is regulated by the Food and Drug Administration (FDA), but the standards can be less stringent compared to tap water regulations.

b. Environmental Impact: Bottled water production and consumption contribute to environmental issues, including plastic waste and carbon emissions from transportation. Tap water, on the other hand, has a smaller environmental footprint as it doesn't involve single-use plastic bottles and transportation over long distances.

c. Cost: Tap water is significantly more cost-effective than bottled water. While tap water is available at minimal cost or as a part of utility bills, the cost of bottled water can quickly add up, especially when consumed regularly.

d. Convenience: Bottled water offers convenience in terms of portability and availability, making it suitable for on-the-go hydration. However, reusable water bottles can offer similar convenience with the added benefit of reducing plastic waste.

It is worth noting that the quality of tap water can vary depending on the location, and some individuals may prefer using home filtration systems to further enhance its taste or remove specific contaminants.

Conclusion: Staying hydrated by consuming an adequate amount of water throughout the day offers a multitude of benefits. From improving physical performance and cognitive function to supporting weight management and digestive health, water plays an indispensable role in maintaining overall well-being. By recognizing the significance of hydration and incorporating sufficient water intake into our daily routines, we can harness these benefits and optimize our health and vitality. Additionally, staying hydrated is a simple yet powerful habit that can have a profound impact on our quality of life, and making informed choices about water consumption and understanding its benefits can contribute to maintaining a healthy lifestyle.

CHAPTER SEVEN

Sugar and its Impact on the Black Community

- Impacts of sugar on diets
- Sugar and chronic diseases
- Disparities in access and Marketing
- Cultural Factors and Sugar consumption
- Vegan "Sugar Alternatives"

This chapter provides a comprehensive understanding of the impact of sugar on the health of the Black community, along with insights into potential solutions to address this issue. Excessive sugar consumption has become a significant concern within the Black community. By understanding the effects of sugar on health and raising awareness, individuals can make informed choices to improve their well-being. Full disclosure this is an area I struggle with even today.

- **Sugar and Chronic Diseases:** High sugar intake has been consistently linked to an increased risk of chronic diseases, including obesity, type 2 diabetes, cardiovascular disease, and certain cancers. Unfortunately, the Black community experiences a higher burden of these conditions compared to other racial and ethnic groups. Studies have shown that too much of sugar consumption is associated with higher rates of obesity and related health issues in these populations, contributing to the health disparities prevalent within the Black community.

- **Disparities in Access and Marketing:** Access to healthier food options is often limited in Black communities, resulting in a reliance on cheaper, processed foods high in added sugars. This lack of access to fresh, nutritious foods is known as a food desert. Moreover, there are disparities in food marketing practices, with sugary products often being heavily promoted in Black communities. This targeted marketing, combined with limited access to healthier alternatives, creates an environment that encourages higher sugar consumption and subsequently leads to adverse health outcomes.

- **Cultural Factors and Sugar Consumption:** Cultural factors play a role in sugar consumption within the Black community. Traditional foods and beverages that are culturally significant may be high in added sugars. Recognizing and preserving cultural practices is essential, but there is also a need to balance promoting healthier alternatives and reducing overall sugar intake. Culturally tailored nutrition education programs can help individuals make informed choices while embracing their cultural heritage.

- **Addressing the Issue:** To mitigate the health implications of sugar in the Black community, a multifaceted approach is needed. Strategies should focus on increasing access to affordable, nutritious foods, particularly in underserved areas. This includes initiatives such as community gardens, farmers' markets, and collaborations with local farmers. Nutrition education programs should be culturally sensitive and emphasize reducing sugar intake. Additionally, implementing policies to reduce sugar consumption, such as sugar taxes and restrictions on marketing unhealthy foods to children can have a positive impact. Community-based initiatives, including grassroots campaigns and collaborations with local organizations are also crucial for raising awareness and advocating for healthier food environments.

Vegan "Sugar Alternatives"

When using these vegan sugar alternatives, keep in mind that they may affect the taste, texture, and moisture content of your recipes. It's a good idea to experiment and adjust the quantities according to your preference.

- **Maple Syrup:** Maple syrup is a natural sweetener derived from the sap of maple trees. It adds a rich flavor to recipes and can be used as a substitute for sugar in baking, beverages, and dressings. Use about 3/4 cup of maple syrup for every cup of sugar and reduce the liquid in the recipe accordingly.

- **Agave Nectar:** Agave nectar is a sweetener derived from the agave plant. It is sweeter than sugar, so you'll need to use less of it. Agave nectar is commonly used in baking, sauces, and beverages. Use about 2/3 cup of agave nectar for every cup of sugar and reduce the liquid in the recipe.

- **Coconut Sugar:** Coconut sugar is made from the sap of coconut palm flowers. It has a similar taste to brown sugar and can be used as a 1:1 replacement in most recipes. Coconut sugar works well in baking, sauces, and desserts.

- **Date Sugar:** Date sugar is made from dried, ground dates. It retains the fiber and nutrients of the fruit, making it a healthier alternative to refined sugar. Date sugar can be used in baking and as a topping for cereals and desserts. Keep in mind that date sugar doesn't dissolve easily, so it may not work well in recipes that require a smooth texture.

- **Stevia:** Stevia is a plant-based sweetener extracted from the leaves of the stevia plant. It is highly concentrated, so a little goes a long way. Stevia is available in powdered or liquid form and can be used in various recipes. Be mindful of the aftertaste, as some people find it slightly bitter.

- **Monk Fruit Sweetener:** Monk fruit sweetener is derived from the monk fruit and has become a popular alternative to sugar. It is highly sweet but doesn't contain any calories or carbohydrates. Monk fruit sweetener can be used as a substitute for sugar in

CHAPTER EIGHT

Food Labels

- Decoding the label
- Understanding serving sizes
- Ingredients List
- Nutrition Facts
- Spotting Hidden Sugars and Sodium
- Allergens and Special Dietary Needs
- Navigating Marketing Claims

Decoding the Label: The Importance of Reading Food Labels In the quest for healthier eating, one crucial tool at our disposal is the ability to decipher the information presented on food labels. In this chapter, we delve into the importance of reading food labels and understanding the valuable insights they provide. By mastering the art of label reading, we can make informed choices that align with our goals for nourishing our bodies and promoting overall well-being.

Understanding Serving Sizes: Food labels contain essential information about serving sizes, which serve as a reference point for understanding the nutritional content of a product. We explore the significance of serving sizes, how they impact calorie intake, and the importance of portion control in maintaining a healthy diet.

Ingredients List: The ingredients list is a window into the composition of a food product. We discuss the significance of this section and the importance of being aware of potentially harmful or undesirable ingredients, such as artificial additives, excessive sugars, unhealthy fats, and preservatives. By familiarizing ourselves with common ingredient names and their implications, we can make more informed choices about the foods we consume.

Nutrition Facts: The nutrition facts panel is a treasure trove of information, offering insights into the macronutrients (carbohydrates, proteins, and fats), micronutrients (vitamins and minerals), and other key components of a food product. We dive into the significance of these nutrients, their recommended daily intake, and how to interpret the percentages provided on the label.

Spotting Hidden Sugars and Sodium: The presence of hidden sugars and excessive sodium in processed foods has been a growing concern. We shed light on the various names for added sugars and high sodium content, providing strategies to identify and reduce consumption of these potentially harmful components.

Allergens and Special Dietary Needs: For individuals with specific dietary needs or food allergies, understanding and accurately interpreting allergen labeling is crucial. We explore common allergens, cross-contamination risks, and the importance of reading labels to ensure the safety and well-being of those with dietary restrictions.

Navigating Marketing Claims: Food packaging often features enticing marketing claims, such as "low-fat," "all-natural," or "organic." Do your research and evaluate these claims and distinguish between true nutritional benefits and mere marketing strategies. By being informed consumers, we can make choices that align with our individual health goals.

Conclusion: Reading food labels empowers us to make conscious and informed decisions about the foods we consume. By understanding serving sizes, ingredients, nutrition facts, hidden sugars, and allergen information, we can navigate the complexities of the modern food industry and make choices that prioritize our health and well-being. In the journey to healthier eating for the Black community, the ability to decode food labels is an invaluable tool that equips us with the knowledge to nourish our bodies and nurture our roots.

CHAPTER NINE

What is The Vegan Lifestyle?

- Defining Veganism and its core principles
- Veganism as a compassionate choice for animals and the environment
- Dispelling misconceptions about Veganism
- The intersectionality of Veganism and Social Justice

Veganism is a lifestyle that seeks to avoid using animal products in all aspects of life, including diet, clothing, and personal care products. It is based on compassion for animals, environmental sustainability, and emotional health. By adopting a vegan lifestyle, individuals can contribute to reducing animal suffering and exploitation. Animal agriculture has significant environmental impacts, including greenhouse gas emissions, deforestation, and water pollution. Choosing plant-based alternatives help mitigate these issues.

There are several misconceptions about veganism, such as the belief that a vegan diet lacks essential nutrients or that it is expensive and inaccessible. This chapter aims to address these misconceptions and provide evidence-based information about the health and environmental benefits of a vegan lifestyle.

Veganism intersects with social justice issues, including racial and economic disparities. By embracing Veganism, individuals can advocate for equitable access to nutritious foods and challenge the systems perpetuating food injustices within marginalized communities.

Vegan Cooking Techniques for Beginners

These cooking techniques are just the beginning, and as you gain confidence and experience, you can explore more advanced methods. Experimenting with different flavors, seasonings, and ingredients will help you create delicious and satisfying vegan meals that you can enjoy every day.

- **Sautéing:** Sautéing involves cooking food quickly in a small amount of oil over medium to high heat. It's a versatile technique that works well for cooking vegetables, tofu, and tempeh. Simply heat oil in a skillet, add your ingredients, and stir them frequently until they're tender and slightly browned.

- **Roasting:** Roasting is a great way to bring out the natural flavors and textures of vegetables. Preheat your oven, toss your vegetables with a little oil and seasonings, then spread them out on a baking sheet. Roast them at a high temperature until they're caramelized and golden brown.

- **Stir-Frying:** Stir-frying is a quick and flavorful cooking method that involves cooking small pieces of food in a hot pan with minimal oil. Heat oil in a wok or skillet, add your vegetables and protein, and stir them constantly over high heat until they're cooked through but still crisp.

- **Steaming:** Steaming is a gentle cooking technique that helps retain the nutrients and natural flavors of vegetables, grains, and tofu. Place your ingredients in a steamer basket or a colander set over a pot of boiling water. Cover and steam until they're tender and cooked to your desired texture.

- **Blending:** Blending is perfect for creating smoothies, soups, sauces, and dressings. Use a high-powered blender to combine ingredients until smooth and creamy. Experiment with different combinations of fruits, vegetables, plant-based milks, and spices to create your desired flavors and textures.

- **Baking:** Baking is a versatile technique used for making bread, muffins, cookies, and cakes. Replace animal-based ingredients with vegan alternatives like flax eggs (ground flaxseed mixed with water), plant-based milk, and vegan butter or oil. Follow recipes carefully and adjust baking times as needed.

Meal Planning Tips for Beginners

Here are ten helpful meal planning tips for beginners transitioning to a vegan lifestyle:

1. **Plan Ahead:** Set aside some time each week to plan your meals and create a shopping list. This will help you stay organized and ensure you have all the necessary ingredients on hand.

2. **Start Simple:** Begin with basic recipes that require minimal ingredients and preparation. As you gain confidence, you can gradually incorporate more complex dishes into your meal plans.

3. **Batch Cooking:** Prepare larger quantities of food and store leftovers for future meals. This saves time and ensures you always have something readily available when you're short on time or energy.

4. **Choose Versatile Ingredients:** Go for ingredients that can be used in multiple recipes. For example, roasted vegetables can be added to salads, grain bowls, wraps, or pasta dishes, providing flexibility in meal options.

5. **Incorporate Plant-Based Proteins:** Ensure your meals are balanced by including plant-based protein sources such as legumes (beans, lentils, chickpeas), tofu, tempeh, or seitan. These ingredients can be used as a focal point or added to various dishes for extra protein.

6.   **Embrace Whole Foods:** Focus on whole, unprocessed foods like fruits, vegetables, whole grains, nuts, and seeds. These provide essential nutrients and contribute to overall health and well-being.

7.   **Prep in Advance:** Take advantage of free time on weekends or evenings to prep ingredients for the week. Chop vegetables, cook
grains, and prepare dressings or sauces to streamline your cooking process.

8. **Explore International Cuisines:** Experiment with recipes from different cuisines that naturally incorporate plant-based ingredients. Mediterranean, Asian, and Mexican cuisines, for example, offer a wide range of vegan-friendly options.

9. **Keep Snacks Handy:** Stock your pantry with healthy vegan snacks such as nuts, seeds, dried fruits, veggie sticks, or homemade energy bars. Having these on hand can help curb cravings and provide quick, nutritious snacks.

10. **Stay Inspired:** Follow vegan food blogs, watch cooking videos, and explore vegan cookbooks to discover new recipes and stay inspired. This will keep your meals exciting and help you develop a diverse and enjoyable vegan meal plan.

By following these meal planning tips, you can simplify your transition to a vegan diet, save time, and ensure a well-balanced and satisfying culinary experience. Remember to listen to your body's needs and adjust your meal plans accordingly.

CHAPTER TEN

Overcoming Barriers and Adopting a Vegan Lifestyle

- Addressing concerns about cultural identity and traditions.
- Tips for transitioning to a vegan diet gradually
- Vegan cooking and meal planning for beginners
- Finding vegan-friendly restaurants and resources

Addressing concerns about cultural identity and traditions

Transitioning to a vegan lifestyle does not require giving up cultural identity or abandoning traditional dishes. This chapter guides how to adapt and incorporate Veganism while honoring cultural heritage and maintaining a sense of belonging. Some people may find switching to a vegan diet difficult. This section offers practical tips and strategies for a gradual transition, allowing individuals to adjust their diets at a comfortable and sustainable pace.

Exploring vegan-friendly restaurants, online resources, and cookbooks can be accommodating when adopting a vegan lifestyle. Please review the table of contents and resources at the end of the book for information on finding vegan-friendly options and recommends valuable recipe ideas and support resources in Chapter 13.

Cooking vegan meals at home can be enjoyable and cost-effective. This section offers practical advice on vegan cooking techniques, meal planning tips, and suggestions for pantry staples to help beginners navigate their new culinary journey.

Tips for transitioning to a vegan diet gradually

Transitioning to a vegan diet can be overwhelming for some individuals. This section offers practical tips and strategies for a gradual transition, allowing individuals to adjust their diets at a pace that feels comfortable and sustainable. It includes suggestions such as starting with Meatless Mondays, gradually reducing animal product consumption, experimenting with new plant-based recipes, and seeking support from vegan communities or online resources.

Transitioning to a vegan diet gradually can help make the process more manageable and sustainable. Here are some tips to help you ease into a vegan lifestyle:

- **Start with Meatless Meals:** Begin by incorporating more plant-based meals into your week. Choose a few days where you focus on vegetarian or vegan options and gradually increase the frequency over time.

- **Replace Dairy and Eggs:** Begin by finding alternatives for dairy and eggs. Experiment with plant-based milk options like almond, soy, or oat milk. Explore tofu, tempeh, or chickpea flour as substitutes for eggs in recipes.

- **Explore New Recipes:** Embrace the opportunity to try new recipes and explore plant-based ingredients. Look for vegan cookbooks or search online for creative and delicious vegan recipes that align with your taste preferences.

- **Focus on Whole Foods:** Emphasize whole, unprocessed foods such as fruits, vegetables, whole grains, legumes, nuts, and seeds. These foods provide essential nutrients and form the foundation of a healthy vegan diet.

- **Gradually Reduce Animal Products:** Slowly decrease your consumption of animal products over time. For example, if you're used to having meat with every meal, start by having it every other day, then gradually reduce it further until you're comfortable without it.

- **Experiment with Substitutions:** Explore plant-based alternatives for meat and dairy products. Try tofu, tempeh, seitan, or plant-based meat substitutes in your favorite recipes. Replace cheese with vegan cheese alternatives made from nuts or soy.

- **Educate Yourself:** Learn about the nutritional aspects of a vegan diet to ensure you're meeting your body's needs. Understand key nutrients like protein, iron, calcium, and vitamin B12, and explore plant-based sources for these nutrients.

- **Connect with Others:** Join vegan or plant-based communities, either online or in person, to connect with like-minded individuals. They can provide support, advice, and share their experiences, making your transition easier.

- **Be Mindful of Labels:** Read food labels carefully to identify hidden animal-derived ingredients. Familiarize yourself with common non-vegan additives and additives that may have animal origins.

- **Practice Self-Compassion:** Be patient and kind to yourself throughout the transition. It's normal to make mistakes or have setbacks. Remember that every step towards a plant-based lifestyle is a positive one.

By gradually transitioning to a vegan diet, you allow yourself time to adjust to new foods, flavors, and cooking techniques. This approach increases your chances of long-term success and enjoyment on your vegan journey.

Pantry Staples

- **Grains and Legumes:** Rice, quinoa, oats, pasta, lentils, chickpeas, black beans, and other varieties of beans provide a great source of protein, fiber, and essential nutrients.

- **Plant-Based Milk:** Stock up on non-dairy milk options such as almond milk, soy milk, oat milk, or coconut milk for use in recipes, smoothies, or as a dairy milk substitute.

- **Nut Butters:** Peanut butter, almond butter, or cashew butter are versatile ingredients that can be used as spreads, added to sauces, or incorporated into baking and cooking.

- **Cooking Oils:** Olive oil, coconut oil, and vegetable oil are commonly used for sautéing, baking, and dressing salads.

- **Herbs and Spices:** Build a collection of dried herbs and spices to add flavor and depth to your dishes. Some essentials include basil, oregano, cumin, turmeric, paprika, and garlic powder.

- **Condiments and Sauces:** Keep vegan condiments on hand like soy sauce, tamari, vegan mayonnaise, mustard, hot sauce, nutritional yeast, and tahini for flavoring and enhancing various recipes.

- **Nuts and Seeds:** Almonds, walnuts, chia seeds, flaxseeds, and sunflower seeds are great for snacking, adding crunch to meals, or as toppings for salads and smoothies.

- **Canned Goods:** Stock up on canned items like diced tomatoes, tomato paste, coconut milk, and vegetable broth for convenient meal preparation.

- **Whole-Grain Flour:** Consider having whole-grain flours like whole wheat, almond flour, or oat flour for baking purposes.

- **Sweeteners:** opt for natural sweeteners such as maple syrup, agave nectar, or coconut sugar as alternatives to refined sugar.

Finding vegan-friendly restaurants and resources

Exploring vegan-friendly restaurants, online resources, and cookbooks can be immensely helpful Doing a Google search in your area will provide information of vegan friendly restaurants. Below are some highly popular online resources:

There are numerous online resources available to support beginners in their journey towards a vegan lifestyle. Here are some helpful websites and platforms that provide valuable information, recipes, and guidance:

- **Vegan Fo Life** www.veganfolife.com) Showtime, a 58-year-old from the Bay Area who transitioned to a vegan lifestyle at 50. Since then, he's experienced improved sleep, increased energy, clarity of mind, and a lack of sickness or anxiety. My aim is to inspire others to prioritize their health through natural herbs and a healthy vegan lifestyle.

- **The Vegan Society** (www.vegansociety.com) This website offers a wealth of information about veganism, including guides on getting started, nutrition advice, and a collection of delicious vegan recipes.

- **Forks Over Knives** (www.forksoverknives.com) Forks Over Knives provides evidence-based resources, meal plans, and recipes focused on whole-food, plant-based eating. They also offer a mobile app for meal planning and recipe discovery.

- **Minimalist Baker** (www.minimalistbaker.com) This blog specializes in simple, plant-based recipes with 10 ingredients or less, requiring minimal time and effort. It's a great resource for beginners looking for approachable and tasty vegan recipes.

- **Oh She Glows** (www.ohsheglows.com) Oh She Glows features a wide range of plant-based recipes, meal ideas, and helpful cooking tips. The recipes are often accompanied by beautiful food photography.

- **The Plant- Based RD (www.theplantbasedrd.com)** Created by a registered dietitian, this website offers evidence-based information, resources, and meal ideas for those interested in a plant-based diet. It covers topics such as nutrition, health benefits, and practical tips for transitioning to a plant-based lifestyle.

- **Veganuary (www.veganuary.com)** Although primarily known for their January campaign encouraging people to try veganism, Veganuary's website offers a wealth of resources year-round. It includes a starter kit, recipes, meal plans, and a supportive community for beginners.

- **YouTube Channels:** There are several popular vegan YouTube channels that provide cooking tutorials, recipe ideas, and lifestyle tips. Some notable channels include "Pick Up Limes," "Avant-Garde Vegan," "The Happy Pear," and "Sweet Potato Soul."

Instagram: Follow vegan bloggers, influencers, and recipe creators on Instagram for inspiration and recipe ideas. Popular accounts include @iamtabithabrown @queenafua@bryantterry@edgyveggie@sweetpotatosoul@yesbabyilike itraw@veganfoodplug@ahimsavegan @fiyabomb @jonimarienewman

Vegan Apps: Consider downloading vegan-friendly mobile apps like "HappyCow" to locate vegan restaurants and food options in your area, and "Is It Vegan?" to help you identify vegan-friendly products by scanning barcodes.

- **Online Vegan Communities:** Engage with online vegan communities and forums, such as r/vegan on Reddit or vegan Facebook groups. These communities provide support, share experiences, and offer advice for beginners.

Remember to explore these resources, experiment with recipes, and find what works best for you. The online vegan community is supportive and enthusiastic, making it easier to navigate your vegan journey and discover new and exciting plant-based options.

CHAPTER ELEVEN

Addressing Socioeconomic Factors

- Strategies for finding affordable vegan options
- Budget-friendly shopping tips
- Community gardens and urban agriculture initiatives
- Advocacy for food justice and equitable access to nutritious foods
- Online Vegan Food Delivery Meal Services

Eating a vegan diet on a budget is achievable with a little planning, mindful shopping, and creative cooking. It's all about finding affordable sources of plant-based protein, embracing whole foods, and making the most of your resources. This chapter provides practical tips for finding affordable plant-based foods, buying in bulk, and making the most of seasonal produce.

- **Plan Meals and Create a Grocery List:** Plan your meals for the week ahead and create a grocery list based on those meal plans. This will help you avoid impulse buying and ensure you only purchase what you need.

- **Compare Prices and Shop Sales:** Take the time to compare prices between different stores or online retailers. Look for discounts, promotions, and coupons to save money on vegan products.

- **Cook at Home:** Cooking your meals from scratch is generally more cost-effective than relying on pre-packaged or processed vegan foods. Focus on simple recipes using whole plant-based ingredients.

- **Buy in Bulk:** Purchase staple items like grains, legumes, nuts, and seeds in bulk. Buying in larger quantities is often cheaper, and these items have a long shelf life, allowing you to save money in the long run.

- **Cook in Bulk and Freeze:** Prepare larger batches of meals and freeze individual portions for later use. This allows you to have quick and convenient meals on hand, preventing the need for takeout or expensive convenience foods.

- **Embrace Seasonal Produce:** Choose fruits and vegetables that are in season as they tend to be more affordable and flavorful. Farmers' markets and local produce stands can offer great deals on seasonal produce.

- **Focus on Whole Foods:** Center your diet around whole plant-based foods like grains, legumes, fruits, vegetables, and nuts. These items are generally more affordable and provide essential nutrients.

- **Embrace affordable Protein Sources:** Beans, lentils, tofu, tempeh, and seitan are affordable and versatile protein sources. Incorporate them into your meals to meet your nutritional needs without breaking the bank.

- **Check out Discount Stores and Ethnic Markets:** Discount stores, dollar stores, and ethnic markets often offer lower prices on produce, grains, and spices. Take advantage of these options to stretch your budget.

- **Grow your own herbs or vegetables:** If you have space, consider growing your own herbs or even some vegetables. It can be cost-effective and rewarding to have fresh produce right at your fingertips.

- **Utilize Frozen Fruits and Vegetables:** Frozen fruits and vegetables are a budget-friendly option and can be just as nutritious as fresh produce. They also have a longer shelf life, reducing the chances of food waste.

- **DIY Snacks and Staples:** Make your own snacks, such as energy bars, granola, or hummus. It's often more cost-effective to make these items at home rather than buying them pre-made. Look for easy DIY recipes online.

- **Limit Processed and Specialty Vegan Products:** While convenient, processed and specialty vegan products can be more expensive. Reserve them as occasional treats and focus on whole, unprocessed foods as the foundation of your diet.

- **Share Meals with Others:** Consider organizing potluck-style meals with friends or family who are also interested in a plant-based diet. Sharing the cost and effort can make eating vegan more affordable and enjoyable.

- **Don't waste food:** Minimize food waste by properly storing leftovers, using scraps for homemade vegetable broth, and repurposing ingredients creatively. This helps save money and reduces waste.

Remember, with a little planning, smart shopping, and some creativity in the kitchen, you can enjoy a budget-friendly vegan lifestyle without compromising on taste or nutrition.

Community Garden Resources

Urban agricultural programs and community gardens can effectively expand access to fresh produce and foster a sense of belonging.

Below is a list of community garden organizations across the US in cities with large Black populations, remember to check the respective websites or contact local organizations for the most up-to-date information on community gardens in each city, as availability and details may change over time.

- **Atlanta, GA:** Atlanta has a growing community gardening movement. The Atlanta Community Food Bank (acfb.org) supports community gardens and offers resources, workshops, and grants to help establish and maintain gardens. They also provide a directory of community gardens on their website.

- **Baltimore, MD:** Baltimore has a thriving community gardening movement. The Baltimore City Farms Program, operated by the Baltimore Office of Sustainability, oversees community gardens in the city. You can find information on community gardens, including locations and contact details, on their website (baltimorecityfarms.org).

- **Birmingham, AL:** Birmingham has community gardens that promote urban agriculture and community involvement. The Jones Valley Teaching Farm (jvtf.org) is an organization that operates multiple urban teaching farms and community gardens in Birmingham. They offer educational programs and resources for community gardening.

- **Chicago, IL:** Chicago has a vibrant community gardening scene. The Chicago Community Gardeners Association (CCGA) is a great resource for finding community gardens in the city. You can visit their website (chicagocommunitygardens.org) to search for community gardens and learn about various programs and initiatives.

- **Cleveland, OH:** Cleveland has a strong community gardening movement. The Cleveland Seed Bank (clevelandseedbank.org) is an organization that supports community gardens and promotes seed saving. They provide resources, workshops, and information on community gardens in the Cleveland area.

- **Detroit, MI:** Detroit is known for its urban agriculture and community gardens. The Greening of Detroit (greeningofdetroit.com) is a non-profit organization that supports community gardens and urban farming. They offer resources, programs, and a garden directory on their website.

- **Los Angeles, CA:** Los Angeles has a strong community gardening culture. The Los Angeles Community Garden Council (lagardencouncil.org) is a non-profit organization that promotes and supports community gardens. Their website offers a garden locator tool and information about gardening resources and programs.

- **Memphis, TN:** Memphis has community gardens that contribute to the city's local food system. The Memphis Area Master Gardeners Association (memphisareamastergardeners.org) provides resources, support, and information on community gardens and urban gardening programs in the area.

- **Mobile, AL:** Mobile has a growing interest in community gardening. The Alabama Cooperative Extension System (aces.edu) offers resources and information on community gardening, including programs and guidelines for starting and maintaining a community garden.

- **New Orleans, LA:** New Orleans has a vibrant community gardening scene. Organizations like NOLA Green Roots (nolagreenroots.com) promote community gardening and urban farming initiatives in the city. Their website provides information on community gardens and resources for starting a garden.

- **New York, NY:** New York City has numerous community gardens spread throughout its boroughs. The New York City Community Garden Coalition (nyccgc.org) is an organization that supports and advocates for community gardens. They provide resources, information, and a garden directory on their website.

- **Oakland, CA:** Oakland has a strong community gardening community. The City of Oakland's website (oaklandca.gov/topics/community-gardens) provides information about community gardens, including a garden directory and guidelines for starting a new garden.
Jackson, MS: Jackson has several community gardens that promote urban agriculture and community involvement. The Mississippi Urban Forest Council (msurbanforest.com) provides

resources and information about community gardens and urban farming initiatives in the state.

- **Philadelphia, PA:** Philadelphia has a rich network of community gardens. The Pennsylvania Horticultural Society (phsonline.org) is actively involved in supporting community greening initiatives, including community gardens. Their website provides resources, events, and information on finding community gardens in Philadelphia.

- **Washington, D.C.:** Washington, D.C. has a vibrant community gardening scene. The D.C. Department of Parks and Recreation oversees community gardens in the city. They offer information on community garden plots, locations, and how to get involved on their website (dpr.dc.gov/page/community-gardens).

Addressing food injustice requires collective action from individuals, communities, and policymakers. It is essential to advocate for policies that promote equitable access to nutritious foods, especially in underserved communities. This includes supporting initiatives that aim to increase funding for programs and services that address food insecurity and improve access to healthy food options. Advocacy efforts can involve raising awareness about the disparities in food access, engaging with local and national policymakers, and supporting organizations that work towards food justice. By joining forces and advocating for change, we can work towards a more equitable and just food system, ensuring that everyone has the opportunity to access and afford nutritious foods for their well-being and overall health.

Recognizing that not everyone has the time or resources to dedicate to preparing vegan meals from scratch, online vegan food delivery services have emerged as convenient and accessible solutions. These services provide a wide range of plant-based options that cater to different dietary preferences and restrictions. By offering pre-prepared meals or meal kits with easy-to-follow recipes, they help bridge the gap for individuals who are interested in adopting a vegan lifestyle but face time constraints or lack culinary expertise.

Online vegan meal delivery services not only save time but also ensure that individuals can enjoy nutritious and flavorful vegan meals without compromising on taste or convenience. These services often prioritize using high-quality, organic, and sustainable ingredients, promoting not just personal health but also environmental consciousness. With the rise of online vegan food delivery services, embracing a plant-based lifestyle has become more accessible and achievable for individuals seeking to make healthier, sustainable choices in their dietary habits.

Online Vegan Meal Delivery Resources

Please note that availability may vary depending on your location, and it's always a good idea to check the websites of these companies for the most up-to-date information on their offerings and delivery areas.

1. Purple Carrot - www.purplecarrot.com Offers plant-based meal kits delivered to your doorstep.

2. Veestro - www.veestro.com Provides fully prepared vegan meals that can be ordered online and delivered nationwide.

3. Daily Harvest - www.daily-harvest.com Delivers vegan smoothies, bowls, soups, and snacks made with whole, organic ingredients.

4. Green Chef - www.greenchef.com Offers meal kits with vegan options, providing pre-portioned ingredients and easy-to-follow recipes.

5. PlantPure - www.plantpurenation.com Provides whole-food, plant-based frozen meals that are ready to heat and eat.

6. MamaSezz - www.mamasezz.com Offers vegan meal delivery with pre-made meals that are free of gluten, oil, and refined sugar.

7. Hungryroot - www.hungryroot.com Delivers vegan-friendly groceries and easy-to-prepare meal kits customized to your preferences.

8. Splendid Spoon - www.splendidspoon.com Delivers plant-based smoothies, soups, grain bowls, and noodle dishes.

9. Urban Remedy - www.urbanremedy.com Offers vegan meal delivery with organic, ready-to-eat plant-based meals, snacks, and juices.

10. The Vegan Garden - www.thevegangarden.com Provides vegan meal delivery with a variety of meal plans to choose from, including gluten-free and low-carb options.

CHAPTER TWELVE

Benefits of a Vegan Diet

- Improved heart health and deflated risk of cardiovascular diseases
- Weight management and diabetes prevention
- Lowered risk of certain cancers
- Enhanced gut health and improved digestion
- Increased energy levels and improved overall well-being

Numerous advantages for heart health have been linked to a carefully thought-out vegan diet. It can lower blood pressure, reduce the risk of cardiovascular disease, and lower LDL cholesterol levels. Plant-based diets are generally low in saturated fats and high in fiber, antioxidants, and minerals that support cardiovascular health, such as potassium and omega-3 fatty acids. Vegan diets, when focused on whole, unprocessed foods, can support weight management and reduce the risk of obesity. Plant-based diets are also associated with better blood sugar control and a decreased risk of type 2 diabetes.

A plant-based diet high in fruits, vegetables, whole grains, and legumes have been displayed in studies to help lower the chance of developing various malignancies, such as colorectal, breast, and prostate cancer. These foods' phytochemicals and antioxidants are essential for preventing cancer. The fiber content of plant-based diets supports a healthy gut microbiome, aiding digestion and promoting regular bowel movements. A diverse and thriving gut microbiome has various health benefits, including improved immune function and mental well-being. Plant-based diets rich in whole foods provide a wide range of nutrients, vitamins, and minerals that support optimal energy levels and general well-being. A well-nourished body is better equipped to combat fatigue and maintain vitality.

CHAPTER THIRTEEN

Recipes:
Plant-Based Alternatives to
Traditional Black Dishes

Breakfast and Brunch

Sweet Potato Pancakes

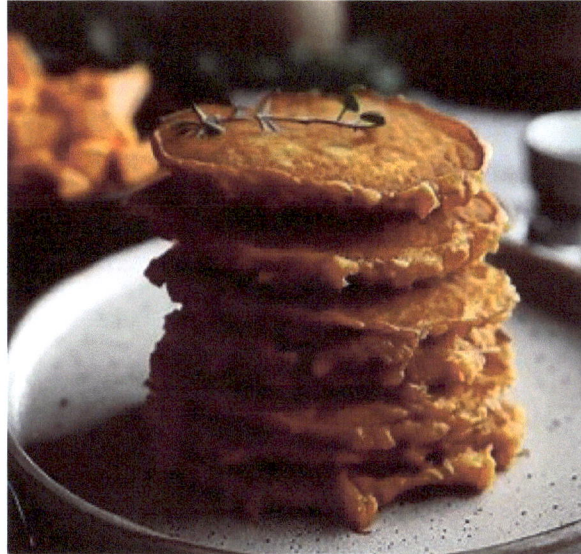

Prep Time: 10 minutes, Cook Time: 15 minutes, Servings: 4

Ingredients

- 1 cup cooked and mashed sweet potatoes (about 2 medium sweet potatoes)
- 1 1/2 cups all-purpose flour or whole wheat flour
- 1 tablespoon baking powder
- 1/2 teaspoon ground cinnamon
- 1/4 teaspoon ground nutmeg
- 1/4 teaspoon salt
- 1 1/4 cups unsweetened almond milk (or any non-dairy milk)
- 1 tablespoon ground flaxseed mixed with 3 tablespoons water (flaxseed egg)
- 1 tablespoon coconut oil or vegetable oil, plus more for cooking
- Optional toppings: maple syrup
- Chopped pecans, sliced bananas, or fresh berries

Instructions

1. In a small bowl, prepare the flaxseed egg by mixing together the ground flaxseed and water. Set aside to thicken for about 5 minutes.
2. In a large mixing bowl, combine the mashed sweet potatoes, flour, baking powder, cinnamon, nutmeg, and salt. Mix well to combined
3. Add the almond milk, flaxseed egg, and coconut oil to the bowl. Stir until all the ingredients are well incorporated, but be careful not to overmix. The batter should be thick but pourable. If it's too thick, you can add a little more almond milk to achieve the desired consistency.
4. Heat a non-stick skillet or griddle over medium heat. Lightly grease the surface with coconut oil or vegetable oil.
5. Using a 1/4 cup measuring cup, scoop the batter onto the skillet to form pancakes. Cook until bubbles form on the surface, then flip and cook for another 1-2 minutes until golden brown.
6. Repeat the process with the remaining batter, adding more oil to the skillet as needed.
7. Serve the sweet potato pancakes warm with your choice of toppings, such as maple syrup, chopped pecans, sliced bananas, or fresh berries.

Soulful Vegan Bacon, Eggs and Grits

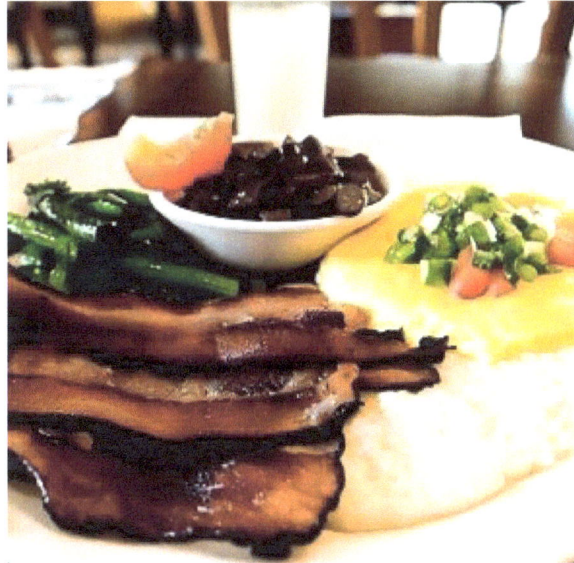

Prep time: 15 minutes, Cook time: 20 minutes, Servings: 2

Ingredients

For the "Bacon"

- 1 block of firm tofu
- 2 tablespoons soy sauce
- 1 tablespoon maple syrup
- 1 tablespoon liquid smoke
- 1/2 teaspoon smoked paprika
- 1/4 teaspoon garlic powder
- 1/4 teaspoon onion powder
- 1/4 teaspoon black pepper
- 2 tablespoons vegetable oil

For the "Eggs"

- 1 block of firm tofu
- 2 tablespoons nutritional yeast
- 1/2 teaspoon turmeric
- 1/2 teaspoon onion powder
- 1/2 teaspoon garlic powder

- 1/2 teaspoon black salt (kala namak) for an eggy flavor
- Salt and pepper to taste

For the Grits

- 1 cup stone-ground grits
- 3 cups water or vegetable broth
- Salt to taste
- Vegan butter or olive oil (optional)

Instructions

1. Prepare the "Bacon"

- Drain and press the tofu to remove excess water. Slice the tofu into thin strips resembling bacon.
- In a bowl, mix together the soy sauce, maple syrup, liquid smoke, smoked paprika, garlic powder, onion powder, and black pepper.
- Marinate the tofu strips in the mixture for at least 15 minutes.
- Heat vegetable oil in a skillet over medium-high heat. Add the marinated tofu strips and cook until crispy and browned on both sides. Set aside.

2. Prepare the "Eggs"

- Drain and press the tofu to remove excess water. Crumble the tofu into a bowl.
- Add nutritional yeast, turmeric, onion powder, garlic powder, black salt, salt, and pepper to the bowl. Mix well to combine.
- Heat a non-stick skillet over medium heat and add the tofu mixture. Cook for about 5-7 minutes, stirring occasionally, until heated through and resembles scrambled eggs. Set aside.

3. Prepare the Grits:

- In a medium saucepan, bring water or vegetable broth to a boil. Add salt to taste.
- Slowly whisk in the grits and reduce the heat to low. Cook for 20-25 minutes, stirring occasionally, until the grits are creamy and tender.

- Remove from heat and add vegan butter or olive oil if desired, stirring to incorporate.

4. Serve:
Plate the creamy grits, top them with the scrambled tofu "eggs,"
- and garnish with the crispy tofu "bacon" strips.
Season with additional salt, pepper, or hot sauce if desired.

-

French Toast

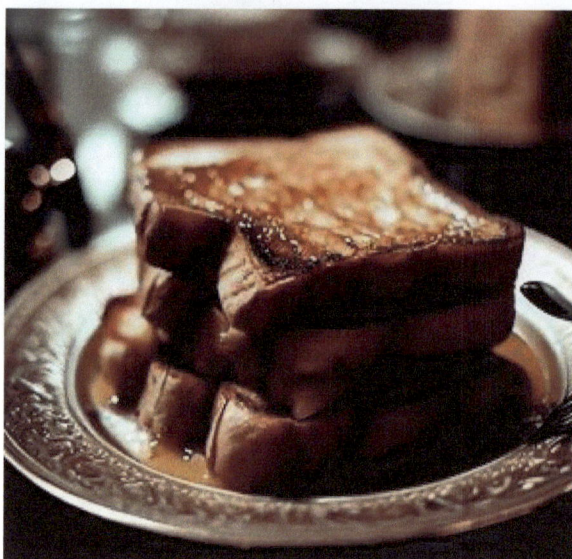

Prep Time: 10 minutes, Cook Time: 15 minutes, Servings: 2

Ingredients

- 4 thick slices of bread
- 1 cup plant-based milk
- 2 tablespoons chickpea flour
- 1 tablespoon nutritional yeast
- 1 teaspoon vanilla extract
- 1/2 teaspoon ground cinnamon
- Pinch of salt
- Maple syrup, fresh fruit, or vegan butter for serving

Instructions

1. Preheat a non-stick skillet or griddle over medium heat.
2. In a shallow bowl, whisk together the plant-based milk, chickpea flour, nutritional yeast, vanilla extract, cinnamon, and salt until well combined.
3. Dip each slice of bread into the batter, coating both sides evenly.
4. Place the coated bread slices onto the preheated skillet or griddle.

5. Cook for 3-4 minutes on each side, or until golden brown.
6. Repeat with the remaining bread slices.
7. Serve the vegan French toast warm with maple syrup, fresh fruit, or vegan butter.

Chickpea Flour Omelet

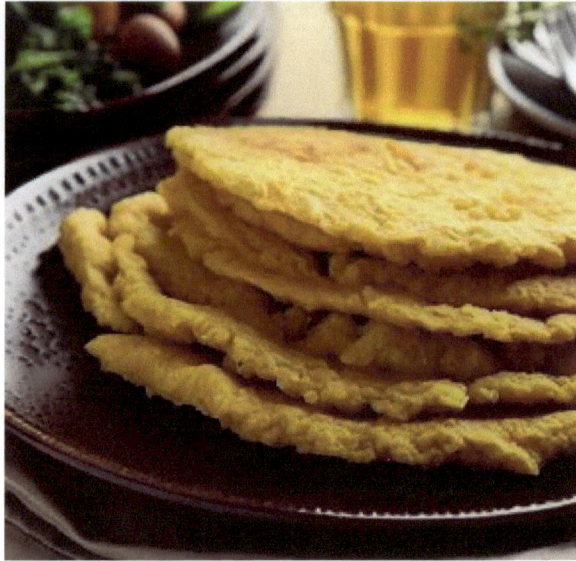

Prep Time: 10 minutes, Cook Time: 10 minutes, Servings: 2

Ingredients

- 1 cup chickpea flour
- ½ cup mushrooms
- 1 cup water
- 2 tablespoons nutritional yeast
- 1/2 teaspoon turmeric
- 1/2 teaspoon baking powder
- 1/2 teaspoon garlic powder
- 1/2 teaspoon onion powder
- Salt and pepper to taste
- Fillings of your choice (e.g., sautéed vegetables, mushrooms, vegan cheese, herbs)

Instructions

1. In a mixing bowl, whisk together the chickpea flour, water, nutritional yeast, turmeric, baking powder, garlic powder, onion powder, salt, and pepper until smooth.
2. Let the batter sit for 5 minutes to thicken.

3. Heat a non-stick skillet over medium heat and lightly grease it.
4. Pour half of the batter onto the skillet and spread it evenly to form a round shape.
5. Cook for 3-4 minutes, or until the edges are set and the bottom is golden brown.
6. Flip the omelet and cook for an additional 2-3 minutes.
7. Repeat with the remaining batter to make a second omelet.
8. Fill each omelet with your desired fillings, fold it in half, and serve hot.

Tofu Scramble

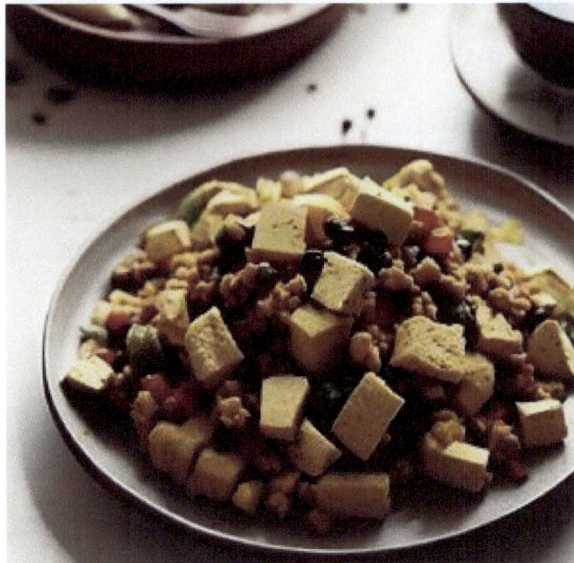

Prep Time: 10 minutes, Cook Time: 15 minutes, Servings: 2-3

Ingredients

- 1 tablespoon olive oil
- 1 small onion, diced
- 2 cloves garlic, minced
- 1 red bell pepper, diced
- 1 block firm tofu, drained and crumbled
- 2 tablespoons nutritional yeast
- 1 teaspoon turmeric
- 1/2 teaspoon cumin
- 1/2 teaspoon paprika
- Salt and pepper to taste
- Fresh parsley for garnish (optional)

Instructions

1. Heat olive oil in a skillet over medium heat.
2. Add onion, garlic, and red bell pepper to the skillet and sauté until softened.

3. Crumble the tofu into the skillet and stir to combine with the vegetables.
4. Add nutritional yeast, turmeric, cumin, paprika, salt, and pepper to the skillet. Mix well to coat the tofu evenly.
5. Cook for about 10 minutes, stirring occasionally, until the tofu is heated through and lightly browned.
6. Taste and adjust seasonings if needed.
7. Garnish with fresh parsley, if desired.
8. Serve the tofu scramble with toast, avocado slices, or your favorite breakfast sides.

Cheesy Grits

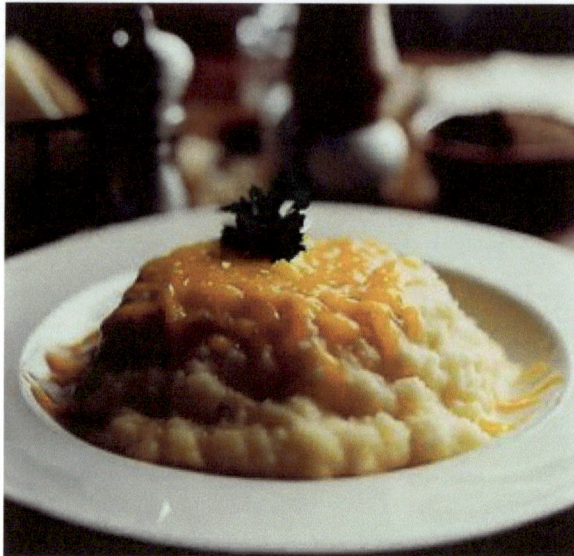

Prep time: 10 minutes, Cook time: 20 minutes, Servings: 4 servings

Ingredients

- 1 cup stone-ground grits
- 3 cups water
- 1 cup unsweetened almond milk (or any non-dairy milk of your choice)
- 1 tablespoon olive oil
- 1 tablespoon nutritional yeast
- 1/2 teaspoon garlic powder
- 1/2 teaspoon onion powder
- 1/2 teaspoon smoked paprika
- Salt and pepper to taste
- Optional toppings: chopped green onions, vegan cheese, hot sauce

Instructions

1. In a medium saucepan, bring the water and almond milk to a boil.

2. Slowly whisk in the grits, reduce the heat to low, and cover the saucepan with a lid. Let the grits simmer for about 15-20 minutes, stirring occasionally to prevent sticking.
3. Once the grits have thickened and become creamy, add the olive oil, nutritional yeast, garlic powder, onion powder, smoked paprika, salt, and pepper. Stir well to combine.
4. Continue cooking the grits for another 5-10 minutes until they reach your desired consistency. If they become too thick, you can add a little more almond milk or water.
5. Taste the grits and adjust the seasonings as needed.
6. Serve the cheesy vegan grits hot in bowls. You can top them with chopped green onions, vegan cheese, and a dash of hot sauce if desired.
7. Enjoy your soulful and cheesy vegan grits!

Hash Browns

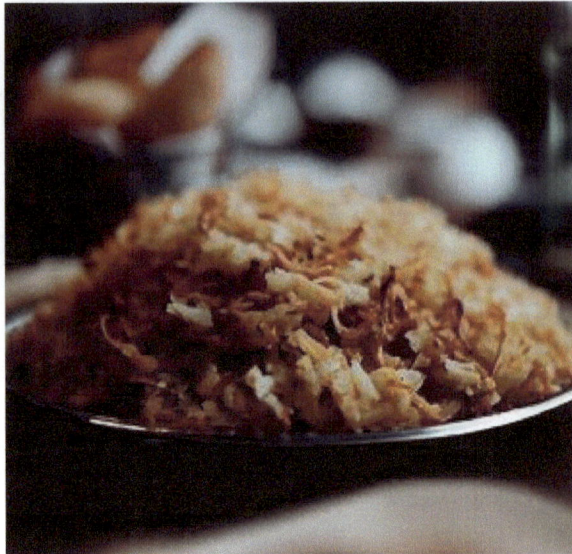

Prep Time: 15 minutes Cook Time: 20 minutes Servings: 4-6 servings

Enjoy the crispy and flavorful vegan hash browns as a tasty addition to your breakfast or brunch!

Ingredients

- 4 medium potatoes, peeled and grated
- 1 small onion, grated or finely chopped
- 2 tablespoons all-purpose flour or chickpea flour
- 1 teaspoon garlic powder
- 1/2 teaspoon onion powder
- 1/2 teaspoon paprika
- Salt and pepper to taste
- 2-3 tablespoons vegetable oil for frying

Instructions

1. Place the grated potatoes in a clean kitchen towel and squeeze out any excess moisture.
2. In a large mixing bowl, combine the grated potatoes, grated onion, flour, garlic powder, onion powder, paprika, salt, and pepper. Mix well until all ingredients are evenly combined.

3. Heat a tablespoon of vegetable oil in a large non-stick skillet over medium heat.
4. Take a handful of the potato mixture and shape it into a patty or a round shape, pressing it firmly together. Place it onto the hot skillet. Repeat with the remaining potato mixture, leaving enough space between each hash brown.
5. Cook the hash browns for about 4-5 minutes on each side, or until they turn golden brown and crispy. You may need to cook them in batches depending on the size of your skillet.
6. Once cooked, transfer the hash browns to a plate lined with paper towels to absorb any excess oil.
7. Serve the vegan hash browns hot as a delicious side dish for breakfast or brunch. They pair well with tofu scramble, vegan sausages, or fresh fruit.

Lentil Curry

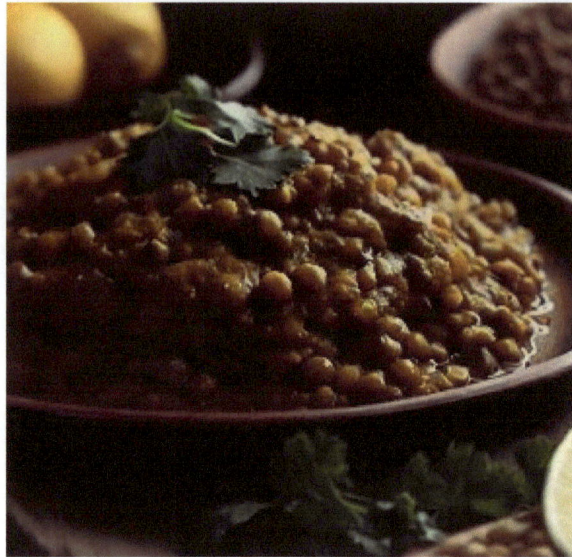

Prep Time: 10 minutes, Cook Time: 30 minutes, Servings: 4

Ingredients

- 1 tablespoon coconut oil
- 1 onion, diced
- 3 cloves garlic, minced
- 1 tablespoon grated ginger
- 2 tablespoons curry powder
- 1 teaspoon ground cumin
- 1/2 teaspoon ground turmeric
- 1 cup dried red lentils, rinsed
- 1 can (14 oz) coconut milk
- 2 cups vegetable broth
- 2 cups chopped vegetables (e.g., carrots, bell peppers, cauliflower)
- Salt and pepper to taste
- Fresh cilantro for garnish (optional)
- Cooked rice or naan bread for serving

Instructions

1. Heat coconut oil in a large pot over medium heat.
2. Add the onion, garlic, and ginger to the pot and sauté until the onion becomes translucent.
3. Stir in the curry powder, cumin, and turmeric, and cook for 1 minute until fragrant.
4. Add the lentils, coconut milk, vegetable broth, and chopped vegetables to the pot.
5. Bring the mixture to a boil, then reduce the heat and simmer for about 20 minutes, or until the lentils and vegetables are tender.
6. Season with salt and pepper to taste.
7. Garnish with fresh cilantro, if desired.
8. Serve the vegan lentil curry over cooked rice or with naan bread.

Lunch & Dinner

Jackfruit Ribs

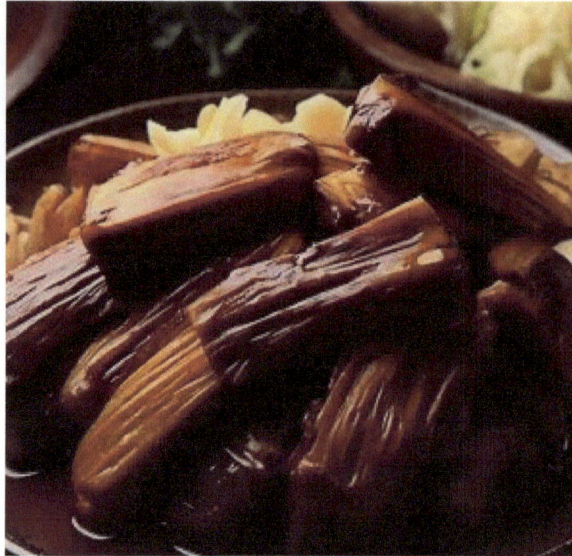

Prep time: 10 minutes, Cook time: 20 minutes, Servings: 4 servings

Ingredients

- 2 cans of young green jackfruit in brine or water (not in syrup)
- 2 tablespoons olive oil
- 1 small onion, finely chopped
- 3 cloves of garlic, minced
- 1/4 cup soy sauce or tamari sauce
- 2 tablespoons tomato paste
- 2 tablespoons maple syrup or agave nectar
- 1 tablespoon liquid smoke
- 1 teaspoon smoked paprika
- 1 teaspoon garlic powder
- 1 teaspoon onion powder
- 1/2 teaspoon ground black pepper
- Salt to taste

For the barbecue sauce:

- 1 cup ketchup
- 2 tablespoons tomato paste
- 2 tablespoons maple syrup or agave nectar
- 2 tablespoons apple cider vinegar
- 1 tablespoon soy sauce or tamari sauce
- 1 tablespoon Dijon mustard
- 2 teaspoons smoked paprika
- 1 teaspoon garlic powder
- 1 teaspoon onion powder
- 1/2 teaspoon ground black pepper
- Salt to taste

Instructions

1. Drain and rinse the jackfruit, then pat it dry. Remove any hard cores or seeds, and shred the jackfruit using your hands or a fork.
2. In a large skillet, heat the olive oil over medium heat. Add the chopped onion and minced garlic, and sauté until they become translucent and fragrant.
3. Add the shredded jackfruit to the skillet and cook for about 5 minutes, stirring occasionally.
4. In a small bowl, whisk together the soy sauce or tamari sauce, tomato paste, maple syrup or agave nectar, liquid smoke, smoked paprika, garlic powder, onion powder, black pepper, and salt.
5. Pour the sauce mixture over the jackfruit in the skillet and stir well to coat. Reduce the heat to low and let the jackfruit simmer in the sauce for about 10-15 minutes, allowing the flavors to blend and the jackfruit to absorb the sauce.
6. While the jackfruit is simmering, prepare the barbecue sauce. In a medium bowl, combine all the barbecue sauce ingredients and whisk until well combined.
7. Transfer the jackfruit mixture to a baking dish and spread it out evenly. Brush the top with a generous amount of barbecue sauce.

8.Bake the jackfruit ribs in the preheated oven for about 20-25 minutes, or until they are slightly caramelized and crispy on the edges.

9. Remove from the oven and let them cool for a few minutes.Serve the soulful vegan jackfruit ribs with additional barbecue sauce on the side and enjoy!

Sliders

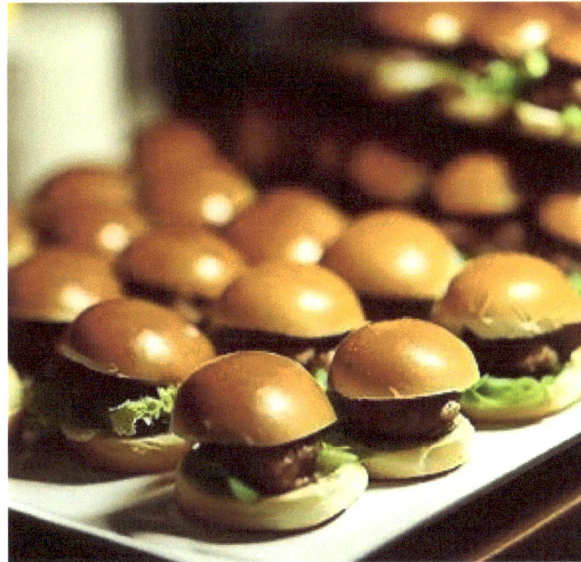

Prep Time: 15 minutes, Cook Time: 25 minutes, Servings: 4-6 servings (12 sliders)

Ingredients

- 1 cup cooked black beans, drained and rinsed
- 1 cup cooked quinoa
- 1/2 cup breadcrumbs
- 1/4 cup finely chopped onion
- 2 cloves of garlic, minced
- 2 tablespoons tomato paste
- 2 tablespoons soy sauce or tamari sauce
- 1 teaspoon smoked paprika
- 1/2 teaspoon ground cumin
- Salt and pepper to taste
- Slider buns

For the toppings:

- Sliced vegan cheese
- Sliced tomatoes
- Lettuce or spinach

- Pickles
- Vegan mayo or sauce of your choice

Instructions

1. In a large bowl, mash the black beans using a fork or potato masher until they are mostly mashed but still have some texture.
2. Add the cooked quinoa, breadcrumbs, finely chopped onion, minced garlic, tomato paste, soy sauce or tamari sauce, smoked paprika, ground cumin, salt, and pepper to the bowl. Mix well to combine all the ingredients.
3. Form the mixture into small patties, about the size of slider buns.
4. Heat a bit of oil in a non-stick skillet over medium heat. Cook the sliders for about 3-4 minutes on each side until they are golden brown and heated through.
5. Assemble the sliders by placing a slider patty on each bun. Add a slice of vegan cheese, sliced tomatoes, lettuce or spinach, and pickles. Spread vegan mayo or your favorite sauce on the top bun.
6. Serve the soulful vegan sliders with your favorite side dishes, such as sweet potato fries or coleslaw.

Sloppy Joes

Enjoy the delicious combination of tangy, smoky, and savory flavors in these vegan sloppy joes!

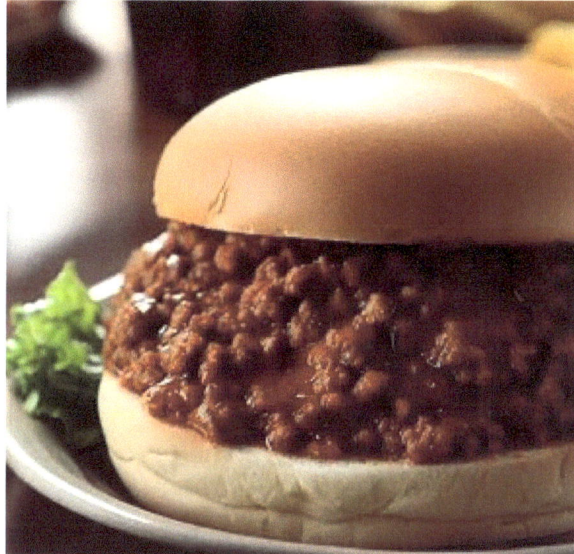

Prep Time: 15 minutes Cook Time: 30 minutes Servings: 4-6 servings

Ingredients

- 1 tablespoon olive oil
- 1 onion, diced
- 1 green bell pepper, diced
- 2 cloves garlic, minced
- 1 cup cooked lentils
- 1 cup cooked black beans, mashed
- 1 cup tomato sauce
- 2 tablespoons tomato paste
- 2 tablespoons maple syrup or molasses
- 2 tablespoons apple cider vinegar
- 1 tablespoon soy sauce or tamari
- 1 teaspoon smoked paprika
- 1 teaspoon chili powder
- 1/2 teaspoon garlic powder
- 1/2 teaspoon onion powder

- Salt and pepper to taste
- Vegan hamburger buns or bread rolls

Instructions

1. Heat the olive oil in a large skillet over medium heat. Add the diced onion and green bell pepper. Sauté until they are softened and lightly browned.
2. Add the minced garlic to the skillet and cook for an additional minute.
3. Stir in the cooked lentils, mashed black beans, tomato sauce, tomato paste, maple syrup or molasses, apple cider vinegar, soy sauce or tamari, smoked paprika, chili powder, garlic powder, onion powder, salt, and pepper. Mix well to combine all the ingredients.
4. Reduce the heat to low and simmer the mixture for 15-20 minutes, allowing the flavors to meld together and the sauce to thicken. Stir occasionally to prevent sticking.
5. Taste and adjust the seasonings as needed, adding more salt, pepper, or spices according to your preference.
6. Toast the vegan hamburger buns or bread rolls, if desired.
7. Spoon a generous amount of the sloppy joe mixture onto each bun or bread roll.
8. Serve your soulful vegan sloppy joes with your favorite side dishes, such as sweet potato fries, coleslaw, or pickles, to complete the meal.

Meatloaf

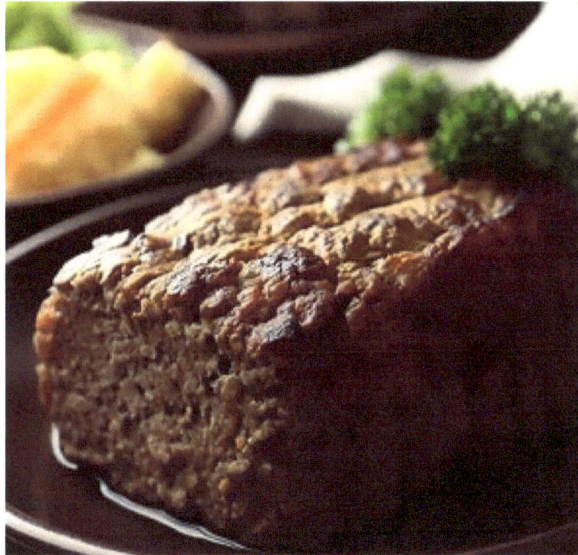

Prep Time: 20 minutes Cook Time: 1.5 hours Servings: 4-6 servings

Ingredients

- 1 cup cooked lentils
- 1 cup finely chopped mushrooms
- 1 cup breadcrumbs
- 1/2 cup finely chopped onion
- 1/2 cup finely chopped bell pepper
- 1/4 cup nutritional yeast
- 2 tablespoons tomato paste
- 2 tablespoons soy sauce or tamari
- 1 tablespoon ground flaxseed mixed with 3 tablespoons water (flax egg)
- 1 teaspoon smoked paprika
- 1 teaspoon garlic powder
- 1 teaspoon onion powder
- 1/2 teaspoon dried thyme
- Salt and pepper to taste

For the Soul Food Twist:

- 1/4 cup barbecue sauce

- 1/4 cup maple syrup
- 1 tablespoon apple cider vinegar
- 1 teaspoon liquid smoke (optional)
- 1/2 teaspoon hot sauce (optional)

For the Glaze:

- 1/4 cup ketchup
- 2 tablespoons maple syrup
- 1 tablespoon apple cider vinegar

Instructions

1. Preheat your oven to 375°F (190°C). Grease a loaf pan or line it with parchment paper.
2. In a large bowl, combine the cooked lentils, chopped mushrooms, breadcrumbs, onion, bell pepper, nutritional yeast, tomato paste, soy sauce or tamari, flax egg, smoked paprika, garlic powder, onion powder, dried thyme, salt, and pepper. Mix well until all ingredients are evenly incorporated.
3. In a separate small bowl, whisk together the barbecue sauce, maple syrup, apple cider vinegar, liquid smoke (if using), and hot sauce (if using).
4. Pour the soul food twist mixture over the meatloaf mixture in the large bowl. Mix everything together until the sauce is well distributed throughout the meatloaf mixture.
5. Transfer the mixture to the prepared loaf pan, pressing it down firmly.
6. In a small bowl, whisk together the ketchup, maple syrup, and apple cider vinegar to make the glaze.
7. Spread the glaze over the top of the meatloaf.
8. Bake the meatloaf in the preheated oven for 40-45 minutes, or until it is firm and the top is slightly caramelized.
9. Remove the meatloaf from the oven and let it cool for a few minutes before slicing and serving.
10. Enjoy your vegan meatloaf with a soul food twist! Serve it with your favorite sides like mashed potatoes, collard greens, or cornbread for a complete soulful meal.

Feel free to adjust the seasonings and flavors to suit your taste preferences. Enjoy the comforting flavors of soul food in this delicious vegan meatloaf!

BBQ Cauliflower Buffalo Wings

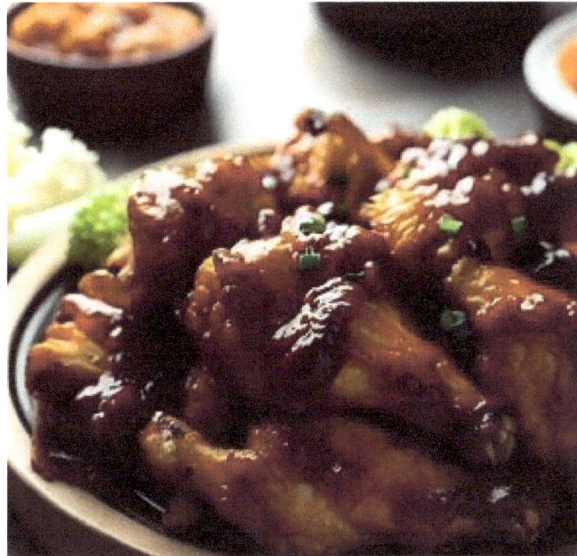

Prep time: 15 minutes, Cook time: 30 minutes, Servings: 4

Ingredients

- 1 head of cauliflower, cut into bite-sized florets
- 1 cup all-purpose flour
- 1 cup plant-based milk (such as almond milk or soy milk)
- 1 teaspoon garlic powder
- 1 teaspoon smoked paprika
- 1/2 teaspoon salt
- 1/4 teaspoon black pepper

For the buffalo sauce:

- 1/2 cup hot sauce (such as Frank's Red Hot or Sriracha)
- 1/4 cup melted vegan butter or margarine
- 1 tablespoon maple syrup or agave nectar
- 1 teaspoon garlic powder
- 1 teaspoon smoked paprika

For serving:

- Vegan ranch or blue cheese dressing
- Celery sticks
- Carrot sticks

Instructions

1. Preheat your oven to 450°F (230°C). Line a baking sheet with parchment paper or lightly grease it.
2. In a large mixing bowl, whisk together the flour, plant-based milk, garlic powder, smoked paprika, salt, and black pepper until you have a smooth batter.
3. Dip each cauliflower floret into the batter, coating it completely, and then shake off any excess batter. Place the coated florets on the prepared baking sheet in a single layer.
4. Bake the cauliflower wings in the preheated oven for about 20-25 minutes, or until they are golden brown and crispy. Flip them halfway through the baking process to ensure even browning.
5. While the cauliflower wings are baking, prepare the buffalo sauce. In a small bowl, whisk together the hot sauce, melted vegan butter or margarine, maple syrup or agave nectar, garlic powder, and smoked paprika until well combined.
6. Once the cauliflower wings are cooked, remove them from the oven and transfer them to a mixing bowl. Pour the buffalo sauce over the wings and toss them gently until they are evenly coated.
7. Return the coated cauliflower wings to the baking sheet and bake for an additional 5-7 minutes to allow the sauce to penetrate and caramelize slightly
8. Remove the cauliflower wings from the oven and let them cool for a few minutes. Serve them with vegan ranch or blue cheese dressing, celery sticks, and carrot sticks on the side.

Fried "Fish"

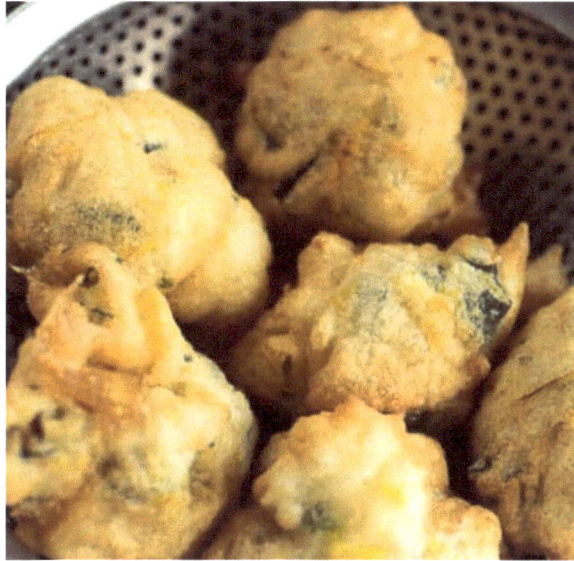

Prep time: 15 minutes Cook time: 15 minutes Servings: based on quantity of fish

Enjoy the crispy and flavorful soul food-inspired vegan fried "fish" as a delicious and satisfying meal

Ingredients

For the "Fish":

- 1 block of firm tofu
- 1 cup unsweetened plant-based milk (such as almond or soy milk)
- 1 tablespoon apple cider vinegar
- 1 cup all-purpose flour
- 1/2 cup cornmeal
- 1 teaspoon paprika
- 1 teaspoon garlic powder
- 1 teaspoon onion powder
- 1/2 teaspoon salt
- 1/4 teaspoon black pepper
- Vegetable oil for frying

For the Tartar Sauce:

- 1/2 cup vegan mayonnaise
- 2 tablespoons sweet pickle relish
- 1 tablespoon lemon juice
- 1 tablespoon chopped fresh dill (optional)
- Salt and pepper to taste

Instructions

1. Press the tofu to remove excess moisture. Cut the tofu into rectangular pieces, resembling fish fillets.
2. In a shallow bowl, combine the plant-based milk and apple cider vinegar. Submerge the tofu pieces in the mixture and let them marinate for at least 30 minutes.
3. In a separate shallow bowl, combine the all-purpose flour, cornmeal, paprika, garlic powder, onion powder, salt, and black pepper.
4. Heat vegetable oil in a deep skillet or frying pan over medium heat. The oil should be about 1 inch deep.
5. Take a tofu piece from the marinade, allowing any excess liquid to drip off, and dredge it in the flour mixture until evenly coated. Shake off any excess flour and carefully place the coated tofu in the hot oil.
6. Fry the tofu for 3-4 minutes on each side, or until golden brown and crispy. Cook in batches to avoid overcrowding the pan.
7. Once cooked, remove the tofu from the oil and place it on a paper towel-lined plate to drain excess oil.
8. In a small bowl, prepare the tartar sauce by combining the vegan mayonnaise, sweet pickle relish, lemon juice, chopped fresh dill (if using), salt, and pepper. Mix well.
9. Serve the vegan fried "fish" hot, alongside the tartar sauce and your favorite soul food sides such as collard greens, cornbread, and coleslaw.

Collard Greens with Tempeh

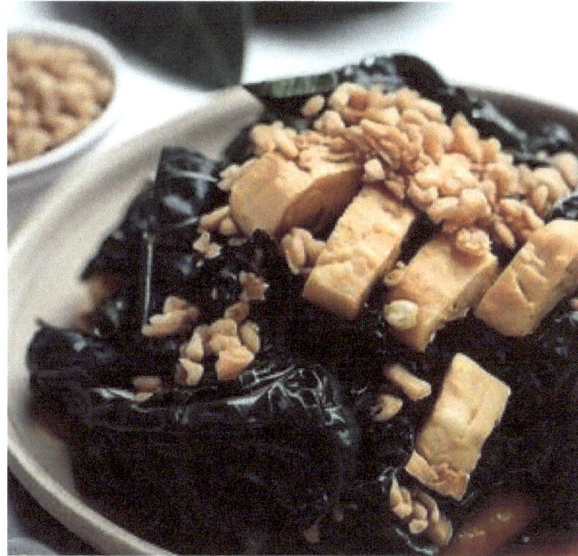

Prep Time: 10 minutes, Cook Time: 25 minutes, Servings: 4

Ingredients

- 1 tablespoon olive oil
- 1 onion, diced
- 3 cloves garlic, minced
- 8 ounces tempeh, crumbled
- 1 teaspoon smoked paprika
- 1/2 teaspoon cayenne pepper (optional)
- 1 bunch collard greens, stems removed and leaves chopped
- 1 cup vegetable broth
- Salt and pepper to taste
- Lemon wedges for serving

Instructions

1. Heat olive oil in a large pan over medium heat.
2. Add the onion and garlic to the pan and sauté until the onion becomes translucent.
3. Crumble the tempeh into the pan and cook for 5 minutes, stirring occasionally.

4. Stir in the smoked paprika and cayenne pepper (if using) and cook for another minute.
5. Add the collard greens and vegetable broth to the pan.
6. Cover the pan and simmer for 15 minutes, or until the collard greens are tender.
7. Season with salt and pepper to taste.
8. Serve the collard greens with tempeh hot, with a squeeze of lemon juice on top.

Lentil Meatballs

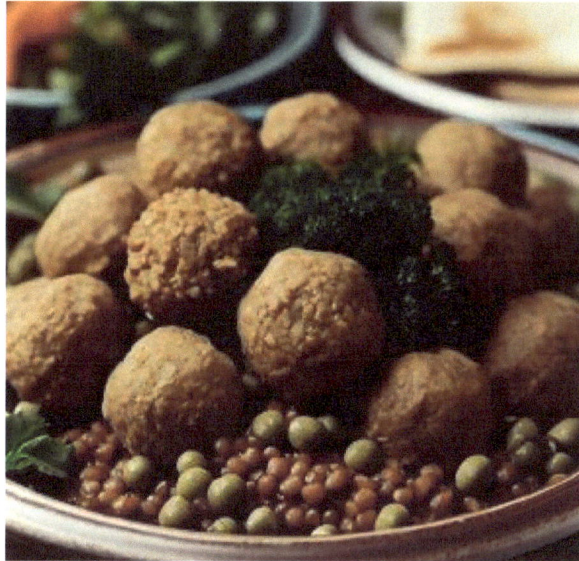

Prep Time: 15 minutes, Cook Time: 25 minutes, Servings: 4

Ingredients

- 1 cup cooked lentils
- 1 cup breadcrumbs
- 1/4 cup nutritional yeast
- 2 tablespoons ground flaxseed mixed with 5 tablespoons water (flaxseed egg)
- 2 tablespoons tomato paste
- 1 tablespoon soy sauce or tamari sauce
- 2 cloves garlic, minced
- 1 teaspoon dried basil
- 1/2 teaspoon dried oregano
- 1/2 teaspoon smoked paprika
- Salt and pepper to taste
- Marinara sauce for serving

Instructions

1. Preheat the oven to 375°F (190°C) and line a baking sheet with parchment paper.
2. In a large mixing bowl, combine the cooked lentils, breadcrumbs, nutritional yeast, flaxseed egg, tomato paste, soy sauce or tamari sauce, garlic, dried basil, dried oregano, smoked paprika, salt, and pepper. Mix well to combine.
3. Roll the mixture into small meatball-sized balls and place them on the prepared baking sheet.
4. Bake the lentil meatballs for 20-25 minutes, or until golden brown and firm.
5. Heat the marinara sauce in a saucepan over medium heat.
6. Once the lentil meatballs are cooked, add them to the marinara sauce and simmer for a few minutes to coat them in the sauce.
7. Serve the vegan lentil meatballs hot, with additional marinara sauce if desired.

Macaroni & Cheese

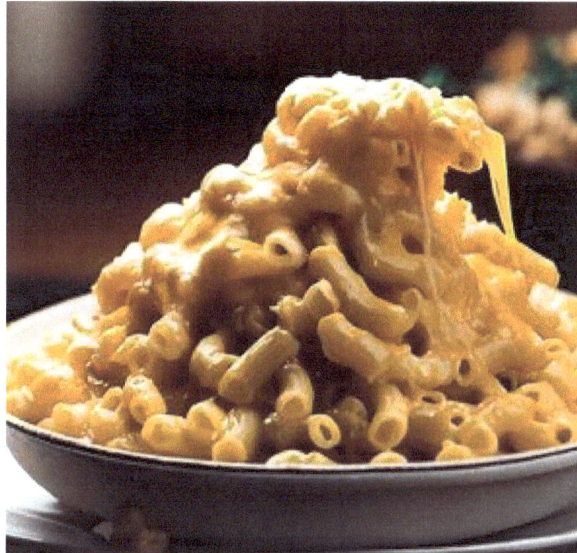

Prep Time: 15 minutes Cook Time: 30 minutes Servings: 4-6 servings

Enjoy the creamy and flavorful vegan macaroni and cheese with a soul food twist!

Ingredients

- 2 cups elbow macaroni (or any pasta of your choice)
- 1 cup raw cashews, soaked in hot water for 1 hour
- 1 1/2 cups vegetable broth
- 1/4 cup nutritional yeast
- 2 tablespoons tomato paste
- 2 tablespoons soy sauce or tamari
- 1 tablespoon Dijon mustard
- 1 tablespoon apple cider vinegar
- 1 teaspoon smoked paprika
- 1/2 teaspoon garlic powder
- 1/2 teaspoon onion powder
- 1/4 teaspoon turmeric (optional, for color)
- Salt and pepper to taste
- 1/2 cup breadcrumbs (optional, for topping)
- 1 tablespoon vegan butter or olive oil (optional, for topping)

Instructions

1. Cook the macaroni according to the package instructions until al dente. Drain and set aside.
2. Drain the soaked cashews and rinse them under cold water.
3. In a blender or food processor, combine the soaked cashews, vegetable broth, nutritional yeast, tomato paste, soy sauce or tamari, Dijon mustard, apple cider vinegar, smoked paprika, garlic powder, onion powder, turmeric (if using), salt, and pepper. Blend until smooth and creamy.
4. Preheat your oven to 350°F (175°C).
5. In a large mixing bowl, combine the cooked macaroni with the cashew cheese sauce. Stir well to coat the macaroni evenly.
6. Transfer the macaroni and cheese mixture to a greased baking dish.
7. If desired, melt vegan butter or heat olive oil in a small saucepan. Stir in the breadcrumbs until coated with the butter or oil. Sprinkle the breadcrumb mixture over the macaroni and cheese.
8. Bake the macaroni and cheese in the preheated oven for 20-25 minutes, or until heated through and the top is golden and crispy.
9. Remove from the oven and let it cool slightly before serving.
10. Serve the soulful vegan macaroni and cheese as a comforting main dish or a side dish. Pair it with collard greens, vegan cornbread, or your favorite soul food sides.

Jollof Rice

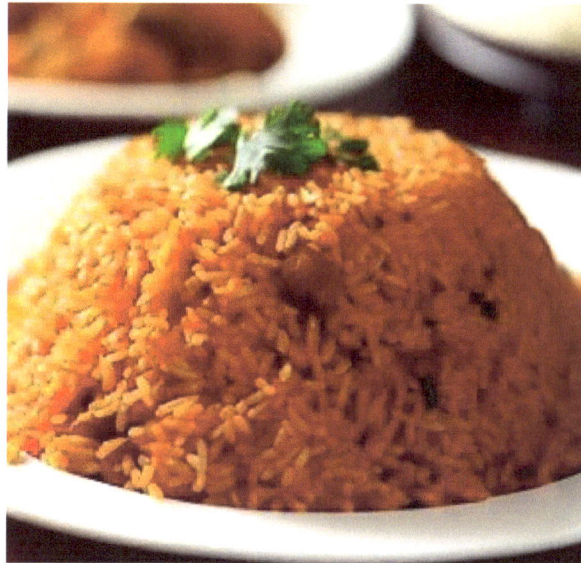

Prep Time: 15 minutes, Cook Time: 40 minutes, Servings: 6

Ingredients

- 2 tablespoons olive oil
- 1 onion, diced
- 3 cloves garlic, minced
- 1 bell pepper, diced
- 1 carrot, diced
- 1 cup diced tomatoes
- 2 cups vegetable broth
- 2 cups long-grain rice
- 1 tablespoon tomato paste
- 1 teaspoon smoked paprika
- 1 teaspoon curry powder
- 1 teaspoon thyme
- 1/2 teaspoon cayenne pepper (optional)
- Salt and pepper to taste
- Fresh parsley for garnish (optional)

Instructions

1. Heat olive oil in a large pot over medium heat.
2. Add the onion, garlic, bell pepper, and carrot to the pot and sauté until the vegetables soften.
3. Stir in the diced tomatoes, vegetable broth, rice, tomato paste, smoked paprika, curry powder, thyme, and cayenne pepper (if using).
4. Bring the mixture to a boil, then reduce the heat to low.
5. Cover the pot and simmer for 25-30 minutes, or until the rice is cooked and the liquid is absorbed.
6. Season with salt and pepper to taste.
7. Fluff the rice with a fork and garnish with fresh parsley, if desired.
8. Serve the vegan jollof rice hot.

Sweet Potato and Black Bean Enchiladas

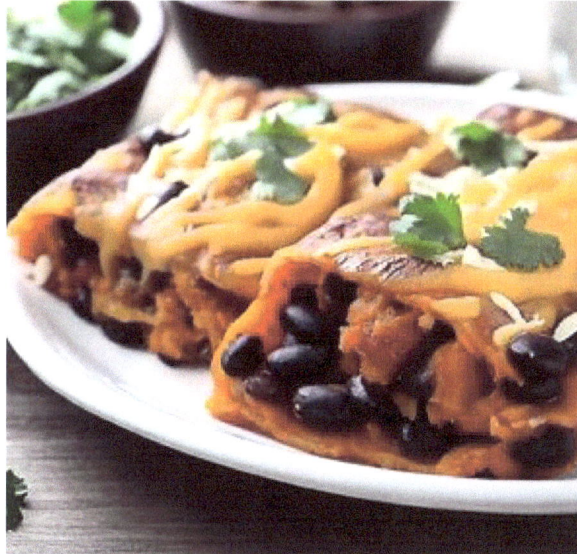

Prep Time: 20 minutes, Cook Time: 25 minutes, Servings: 4

Ingredients

- 2 large sweet potatoes, peeled and cubed
- 1 tablespoon olive oil
- 1 onion, diced
- 3 cloves garlic, minced
- 1 bell pepper, diced
- 1 can (15 oz) black beans, drained and rinsed
- 1 teaspoon ground cumin
- 1/2 teaspoon chili powder
- Salt and pepper to taste
- 8 small tortillas (corn or flour)
- 1 cup enchilada sauce
- Vegan cheese, shredded (optional)
- Fresh cilantro for garnish (optional)

Instructions

1. Preheat the oven to 375°F (190°C) and lightly grease a baking dish
2. Place the sweet potatoes in a steamer basket and steam until tender, about 10-15 minutes.
3. In a large skillet, heat the olive oil over medium heat.
4. Add the onion, garlic, and bell pepper to the skillet and sauté until the onion becomes translucent.
5. Stir in the black beans, cumin, chili powder, salt, and pepper. Cook for another 2-3 minutes, then remove from heat.
6. In a mixing bowl, mash the steamed sweet potatoes.
7. Add the black bean mixture to the mashed sweet potatoes and mix well.
8. Spoon the sweet potato and black bean filling onto each tortilla, then roll them up and place them seam-side down in the prepared baking dish.
9. Pour the enchilada sauce over the rolled tortillas, making sure to cover them evenly.
10. If desired, sprinkle vegan cheese on top.
11. Bake in the preheated oven for 20-25 minutes, or until the enchiladas are heated through and the sauce is bubbling.
12. Garnish with fresh cilantro, if desired.
13. Serve the vegan sweet potato and black bean enchiladas hot.

Jambalaya

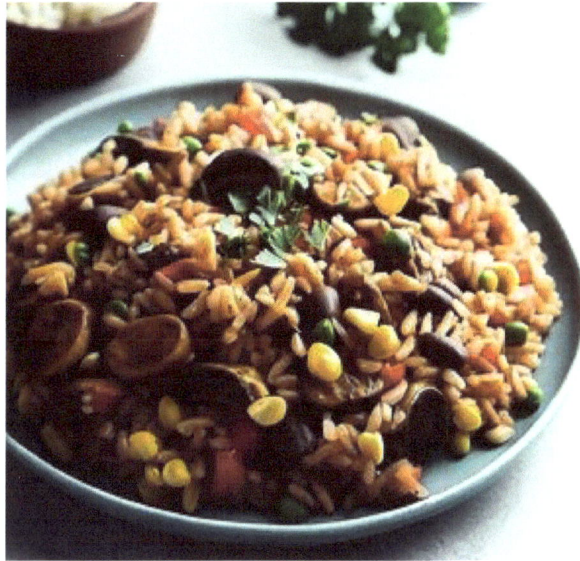

Prep Time: 15 minutes, Cook Time: 40 minutes, Servings: 4-6 servings

Ingredients

- 2 tablespoons vegetable oil
- 1 onion, diced
- 2 bell peppers, diced
- 3 celery stalks, diced
- 4 cloves of garlic, minced
- 1 cup diced tomatoes (canned or fresh)
- 1 cup sliced vegan sausage (such as seitan or plant-based sausage)
- 1 cup diced vegan chicken (such as tofu or plant-based chicken substitutes)
- 2 cups vegetable broth
- 1 cup long-grain rice
- 2 teaspoons Cajun seasoning
- 1 teaspoon smoked paprika
- 1/2 teaspoon dried thyme
- 1/2 teaspoon dried oregano
- 1/4 teaspoon cayenne pepper (adjust to your spice preference)

- Salt and pepper to taste
- Chopped green onions, for garnish

Instructions

1. In a large pot, heat the vegetable oil over medium heat. Add the onion, bell peppers, celery, and garlic. Sauté for about 5 minutes until the vegetables are tender.
2. Add the diced tomatoes, vegan sausage, vegan chicken, vegetable broth, long-grain rice, Cajun seasoning, smoked paprika, dried thyme, dried oregano, cayenne pepper, salt, and pepper. Stir well to combine.
3. Bring the mixture to a boil, then reduce the heat to low. Cover the pot and let the jambalaya simmer for about 20-25 minutes, or until the rice is cooked and the flavors have melded together. Stir occasionally to prevent sticking.
4. Once the rice is cooked, taste the jambalaya and adjust the seasonings if needed.
5. Serve the vegan New Orleans-style jambalaya hot, garnished with chopped green onions.

Shrimp & Chicken Gumbo

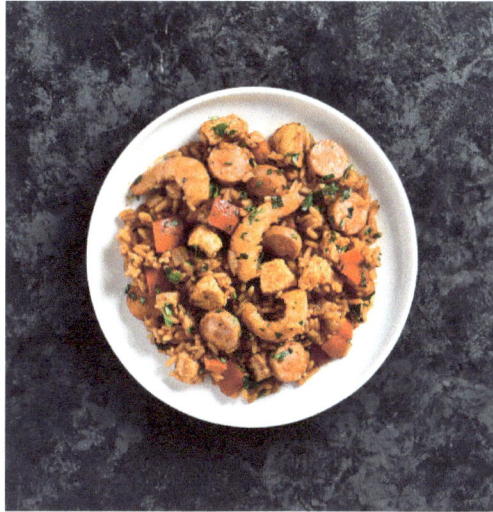

Prep Time: 15 minutes, Cook Time: 30 minutes, Servings: 4-6 servings

Ingredients

- 1 package of vegan chicken strips (such as plant-based chicken substitutes)
- 1 package of vegan shrimp (such as plant-based shrimp substitutes)

For the gumbo:

- 2 tablespoons vegetable oil
- 1 onion, diced
- 2 bell peppers, diced
- 3 celery stalks, diced
- 4 cloves of garlic, minced
- 1 can diced tomatoes
- 4 cups vegetable broth
- 1 cup okra, sliced
- 1 cup sliced vegan sausage (such as seitan or plant-based sausage)
- 1 tablespoon Cajun seasoning
- 1 teaspoon smoked paprika
- 1/2 teaspoon dried thyme

- 1/2 teaspoon dried oregano
- 1/4 teaspoon cayenne pepper (adjust to your spice preference)
- Salt and pepper to taste
- Cooked rice, for serving
- Chopped green onions, for garnish

Instructions

1. Prepare the vegan chicken and shrimp according to the package instructions. This usually involves thawing them and lightly sautéing them in a pan with oil. Set aside.
2. In a large pot, heat the vegetable oil over medium heat. Add the onion, bell peppers, celery, and garlic. Sauté for about 5 minutes until the vegetables are tender.
3. Add the diced tomatoes, vegetable broth, okra, vegan sausage, Cajun seasoning, smoked paprika, dried thyme, dried oregano, cayenne pepper, salt, and pepper. Stir well to combine.
4. Bring the gumbo to a boil, then reduce the heat to low. Cover the pot and let the gumbo simmer for about 20-25 minutes to allow the flavors to meld together.
5. Taste the gumbo and adjust the seasonings if needed.
6. Add the prepared vegan chicken and shrimp to the gumbo, stirring gently to incorporate them without breaking them apart. Allow the gumbo to simmer for an additional 5 minutes to heat the chicken and shrimp through.
7. Serve the soulful vegan chicken, shrimp, and vegetable gumbo hot over cooked rice. Garnish with chopped green onions.

Thanksgiving "Turkey" Dinner

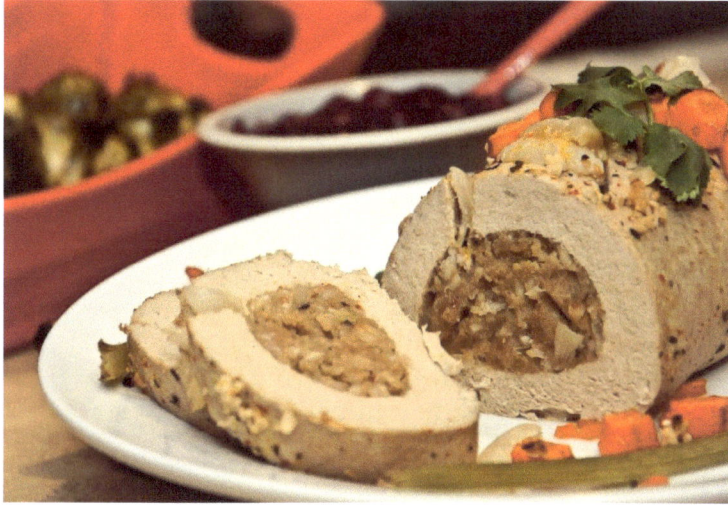

Prep Time: 30 minutes Cook Time: 3-4 hours Servings: 8-12

Main Dish: Vegan Stuffed Seitan "Turkey" Roast

Ingredients

For the Seitan "Turkey":

- 2 cups vital wheat gluten
- 1/4 cup nutritional yeast
- 2 tablespoons chickpea flour
- 1 tablespoon onion powder
- 1 tablespoon garlic powder
- 1 teaspoon smoked paprika
- 1 teaspoon poultry seasoning
- 1/2 teaspoon black pepper
- 1 1/2 cups vegetable broth
- 1/4 cup soy sauce or tamari
- 2 tablespoons tomato paste
- 2 tablespoons liquid smoke
- 2 tablespoons olive oil

For the Dressing:

- 2 cups cubed bread (such as whole wheat or sourdough)

- 1/2 cup diced onion
- 1/2 cup diced celery
- 1/2 cup diced bell pepper
- 2 cloves garlic, minced
- 1 teaspoon dried thyme
- 1 teaspoon dried sage
- 1/2 teaspoon black pepper
- 1/2 cup vegetable broth or water

For the Gravy:

- 2 tablespoons vegan butter or olive oil
- 2 tablespoons all-purpose flour
- 2 cups vegetable broth
- 2 tablespoons soy sauce or tamari
- Salt and pepper to taste

Instructions

1. Preheat your oven to 350°F (175°C). Grease a baking dish or line it with parchment paper.
2. In a large mixing bowl, combine the vital wheat gluten, nutritional yeast, chickpea flour, onion powder, garlic powder, smoked paprika, poultry seasoning, and black pepper.
3. In a separate bowl, whisk together the vegetable broth, soy sauce or tamari, tomato paste, liquid smoke, and olive oil.
4. Pour the wet mixture into the dry ingredients and stir until a dough forms. Knead the dough for a few minutes until it becomes elastic.
5. In a large skillet, melt vegan butter or heat olive oil over medium heat. Add the diced onion, celery, bell pepper, garlic, dried thyme, dried sage, and black pepper. Sauté until the vegetables are tender.
6. In a separate bowl, combine the sautéed vegetables with the cubed bread. Gradually add vegetable broth or water until the dressing is moist but not soggy.

7. Roll out the seitan dough into a rectangular shape on a clean surface. Spread the dressing mixture evenly over the seitan, leaving a small border around the edges.
8. Carefully roll up the seitan, starting from one of the longer sides, to form a log shape. Pinch the ends to seal.
9. Place the seitan log in the greased baking dish and cover it with foil. Bake in the preheated oven for 1 hour.
10. Remove the foil and continue baking for an additional 15 minutes, or until the seitan is firm and golden brown.
11. While the seitan is baking, prepare the gravy. In a saucepan, melt vegan butter or heat olive oil over medium heat. Stir in the all-purpose flour and cook for a minute to form a roux.
12. Gradually whisk in the vegetable broth and soy sauce or tamari. Cook the gravy, stirring constantly, until it thickens. Season with salt and pepper to taste.
13. Once the seitan is cooked, remove it from the oven and let it cool for a few minutes before slicing.
14. Serve the sliced seitan "turkey" roast with the homemade gravy, along with traditional Thanksgiving side dishes like mashed potatoes, roasted vegetables, collard greens, and cornbread for a soulful vegan Thanksgiving dinner.

Black Bean Soup

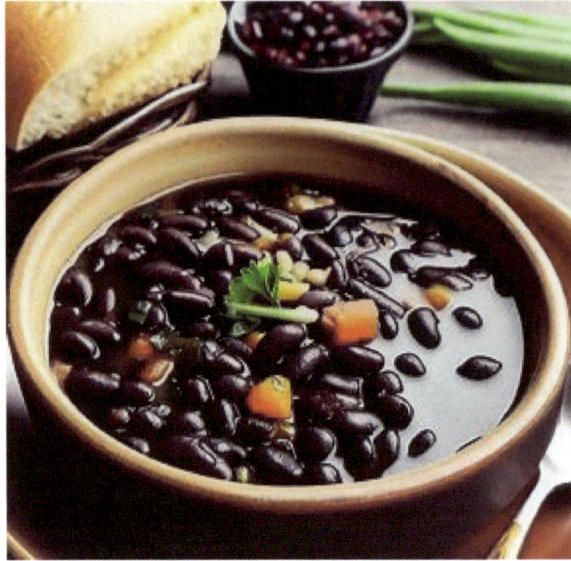

Prep time: 10 minutes, Cook time: 30 minutes, Servings: 4

Ingredients

- 2 tablespoons olive oil
- 1 onion, diced
- 2 bell peppers, diced
- 3 cloves of garlic, minced
- 2 cans black beans, drained and rinsed
- 1 can diced tomatoes
- 4 cups vegetable broth
- 1 tablespoon chili powder
- 1 teaspoon ground cumin
- 1 teaspoon smoked paprika
- 1/2 teaspoon dried oregano
- Juice of 1 lime
- Salt and pepper to taste
- Chopped fresh cilantro, for garnish
- Avocado slices, for garnish

Instructions

1. In a large pot, heat the olive oil over medium heat. Add the onion, bell peppers, and garlic. Sauté for about 5 minutes until the vegetables are tender.
2. Add the black beans, diced tomatoes (with their juice), vegetable broth, chili powder, cumin, smoked paprika, dried oregano, salt, and pepper. Stir well to combine.
3. Bring the soup to a boil, then reduce the heat to low. Cover the pot and let the soup simmer for about 20-25 minutes to allow the flavors to meld together.
4. Use an immersion blender or transfer a portion of the soup to a blender, and blend until smooth. This step is optional, but it helps thicken the soup and create a smoother texture.
5. Stir in the lime juice and taste the soup. Adjust the seasonings if needed.
6. Serve the vegan black bean soup hot. Garnish with chopped fresh cilantro and avocado slices.

Gumbo Soup

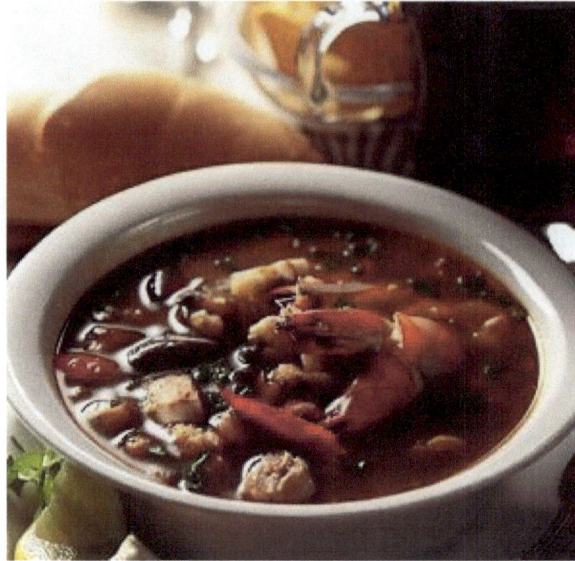

Prep Time: 15 minutes, Cook Time: 45 minutes, Servings: 4-6

Ingredients

- 2 tablespoons vegetable oil
- 1 onion, diced
- 2 bell peppers, diced
- 2 celery stalks, diced
- 3 cloves of garlic, minced
- 1 can diced tomatoes
- 4 cups vegetable broth
- 1 cup okra, sliced
- 1 cup cooked kidney beans
- 1 cup cooked chickpeas
- 1 cup sliced vegan sausage (such as seitan or plant-based sausage)
- 1 tablespoon Cajun seasoning
- 1 teaspoon smoked paprika
- 1/2 teaspoon dried thyme
- Salt and pepper to taste
- Cooked rice, for serving
- Chopped green onions, for garnish

Instructions

1. In a large pot, heat the vegetable oil over medium heat. Add the onion, bell peppers, celery, and garlic. Sauté for about 5 minutes until the vegetables are tender.
2. Add the diced tomatoes, vegetable broth, okra, kidney beans, chickpeas, vegan sausage, Cajun seasoning, smoked paprika, dried thyme, salt, and pepper. Stir well to combine.
3. Bring the soup to a boil, then reduce the heat to low. Cover the pot and let the soup simmer for about 20-25 minutes to allow the flavors to meld together.
4. Taste the soup and adjust the seasonings if needed.
5. Serve the vegan gumbo soup hot over cooked rice. Garnish with chopped green onions.

Butternut Squash Soup

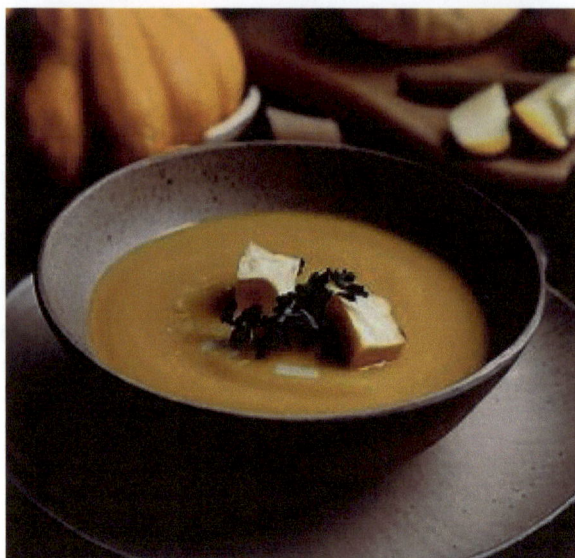

Prep Time: 15 minutes, Cook Time: 30 minutes, Servings: 4

Ingredients

- 1 tablespoon olive oil
- 1 onion, diced
- cloves garlic, minced
- 1 medium butternut squash, peeled, seeded, and cubed
- 3 carrots, peeled and chopped
- 4 cups vegetable broth
- 1 teaspoon ground cumin
- 1/2 teaspoon ground cinnamon
- 1/4 teaspoon nutmeg
- Salt and pepper to taste
- Coconut milk for garnish (optional)
- Fresh parsley or chives for garnish (optional)

Instructions

Heat olive oil in a large pot over medium heat.

1. Add the onion and garlic to the pot and sauté until the onion becomes translucent.

2. Add the butternut squash, carrots, vegetable broth, cumin, cinnamon, and nutmeg to the pot.
3. Bring the mixture to a boil, then reduce the heat and simmer for about 20-25 minutes, or until the butternut squash and carrots are tender.
4. Use an immersion blender or transfer the soup to a blender to puree until smooth.
5. Season with salt and pepper to taste.
6. Serve the vegan butternut squash soup hot, garnished with a drizzle of coconut milk and fresh parsley or chives, if desired.

Fiesta Taco Bowl

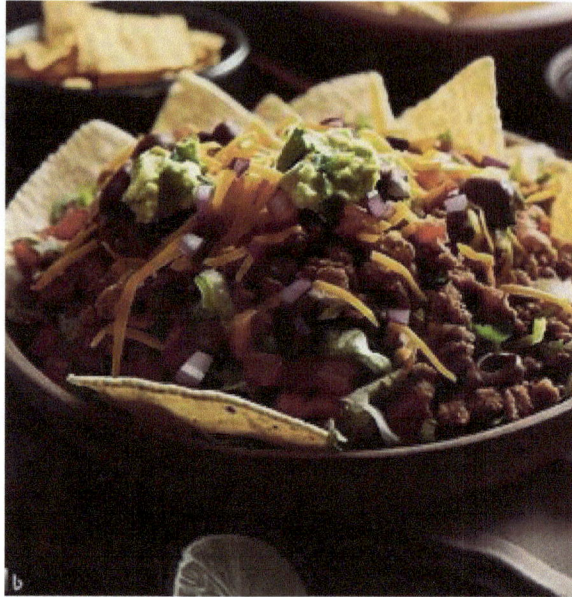

Prep Time: 20 minutes Cook Time: 30 minutes Servings: 4-6 servings

Ingredients

For the Stewed Black Beans:

- 1 can (15 ounces) black beans, drained and rinsed
- 1 small onion, finely chopped
- 2 cloves of garlic, minced
- 1 teaspoon cumin powder
- 1 teaspoon paprika
- 1/2 teaspoon chili powder
- Salt and pepper to taste

For the Grilled Corn:

- 2 ears of corn, husked
- 1 tablespoon olive oil
- Salt and pepper to taste

For the Pico de Gallo:

- 2 tomatoes, diced

- 1/2 red onion, finely chopped
- 1 jalapeno pepper, seeds removed and finely chopped
- Juice of 1 lime
- 2 tablespoons fresh cilantro, chopped
- Salt and pepper to taste

For the Chipotle Aioli:

- 1/2 cup vegan mayonnaise
- 1-2 chipotle peppers in adobo sauce, finely chopped
- 1 tablespoon lime juice
- Salt to taste

For the Fiesta Taco Bowl:

- Cooked rice (brown, white, or cauliflower rice)
- Shredded lettuce or baby spinach
- Sliced avocado
- Sliced radishes (optional)
- Fresh cilantro, chopped (for garnish)

Instructions

1. Start by preparing the stewed black beans. In a saucepan, heat a little bit of olive oil over medium heat. Add the chopped onion and minced garlic, sauté until fragrant and translucent.
2. Add the drained black beans, cumin powder, paprika, chili powder, salt, and pepper to the saucepan. Stir well to combine all the ingredients. Allow the beans to simmer on low heat for about 10-15 minutes, stirring occasionally.
3. While the beans are stewing, preheat your grill or grill pan to medium-high heat. Brush the corn with olive oil and season with salt and pepper. Grill the corn until slightly charred, turning occasionally for even cooking. Remove from the grill and let it cool slightly. Once cooled, cut the kernels off the cob.
4. To make the pico de gallo, combine diced tomatoes, red onion, jalapeno pepper, lime juice, chopped cilantro, salt, and pepper in a bowl. Mix well and set aside.

5. For the chipotle aioli, in a small bowl, whisk together the vegan mayonnaise, chopped chipotle peppers, lime juice, and salt until well combined. Adjust the amount of chipotle peppers according to your desired level of spiciness.
6. Assemble your Fiesta Taco Bowl: Start with a base of cooked rice in a bowl. Top it with the stewed black beans, grilled corn, pico de gallo, sliced avocado, shredded lettuce or baby spinach, and sliced radishes if desired.
7. Drizzle the chipotle aioli over the top of the bowl. Garnish with fresh cilantro.
8. Serve your vegan Fiesta Taco Bowl immediately and enjoy!

Curry Chickpea Ragu Bowl

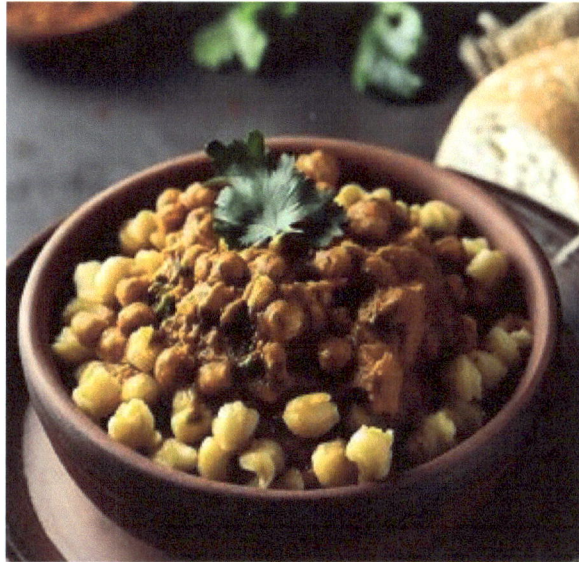

Prep Time: 20 minutes Cook Time: 40 minutes Servings: 4 servings

Ingredients

For the Curry Chickpea Ragu:

- 2 tablespoons olive oil
- 1 small onion, finely chopped
- 2 cloves of garlic, minced
- 1 red bell pepper, diced
- 1 carrot, diced
- 1 teaspoon curry powder
- 1 teaspoon ground cumin
- 1 teaspoon paprika
- 1/2 teaspoon turmeric
- 1 can (15 ounces) chickpeas, drained and rinsed
- 1 can (14 ounces) diced tomatoes
- 1 cup vegetable broth
- Salt and pepper to taste

For the Bowl:

- Cooked rice or quinoa

- Steamed or sautéed vegetables (such as broccoli, cauliflower, or bell peppers)
- Fresh cilantro, chopped (for garnish)

Instructions

1. Heat olive oil in a large skillet over medium heat. Add the chopped onion and minced garlic, and sauté until fragrant and translucent.
2. Add the diced red bell pepper and carrot to the skillet. Sauté for a few minutes until the vegetables start to soften.
3. In a small bowl, combine the curry powder, ground cumin, paprika, and turmeric. Add the spice mixture to the skillet and stir to coat the vegetables.
4. Add the drained and rinsed chickpeas, diced tomatoes (with their juices), and vegetable broth to the skillet. Stir well to combine all the ingredients.
5. Reduce the heat to low and let the mixture simmer for about 15-20 minutes, stirring occasionally. The flavors will meld together, and the ragu will thicken slightly.
6. Season the ragu with salt and pepper to taste. Adjust the spices if desired.
7. Assemble your Curry Chickpea Ragu Bowl: Start with a base of cooked rice or quinoa in a bowl. Top it with a generous scoop of the curry chickpea ragu.
8. Add steamed or sautéed vegetables of your choice to the bowl. You can use broccoli, cauliflower, bell peppers, or any other vegetables you prefer.
9. Garnish with fresh chopped cilantro.
10. Serve your vegan Curry Chickpea Ragu Bowl hot and enjoy!

Kale Cesar Salad Bowl

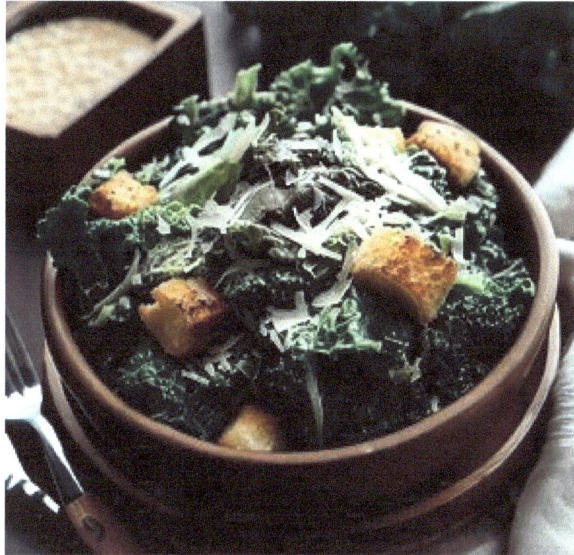

Prep Time: 20 minutes Cook Time: - Servings: 4 servings

Enjoy your delicious and nutritious Kale Caesar salad! Feel free to adjust the quantities of ingredients according to your taste preferences.

Ingredients

- Fresh kale leaves, washed and torn into bite-sized pieces
- Cucumber, thinly sliced
- Carrots, grated or julienned
- Cherry tomatoes, halved
- Vegan Parmesan cheese (store-bought or homemade)
- Vegan crostini (store-bought or homemade)

For the Dressing:

- 1/4 cup vegan mayonnaise
- 2 tablespoons lemon juice
- 2 tablespoons nutritional yeast
- 1 tablespoon Dijon mustard
- 2 cloves garlic, minced
- Salt and pepper to taste

Instructions

1. In a large bowl, combine the kale, sliced cucumber, grated carrots, and cherry tomatoes.
2. Prepare the dressing by whisking together the vegan mayonnaise, lemon juice, nutritional yeast, Dijon mustard, minced garlic, salt, and pepper in a small bowl.
3. Drizzle the dressing over the kale and vegetable mixture. Toss well to coat the ingredients evenly.
4. Sprinkle vegan Parmesan cheese over the salad and gently toss again.
5. Serve the Power Kale Caesar salad in individual bowls or plates, and garnish with vegan crostini.

BBQ Jackfruit Pizza

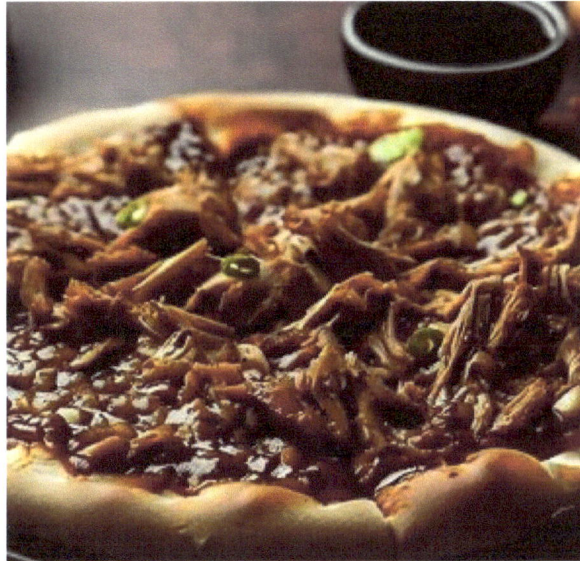

Prep Time: 20 minutes, Cook Time: 30 minutes, Servings: 4-6

Ingredients

- 1 vegan pre-made pizza crust (check for vegan options)
- 1 can of young jackfruit in brine, drained and rinsed
- 1/2 cup BBQ sauce (check for vegan-friendly)
- 1/2 red onion, thinly sliced
- 1/2 cup sliced bell peppers (any color)
- 1 cup vegan cheese (such as vegan mozzarella or cheddar)
- Fresh cilantro, chopped (for garnish)

Instructions

1. Preheat the oven according to the pizza crust package instructions.
2. In a pan, sauté the jackfruit for a few minutes until it starts to soften. Add the BBQ sauce and cook for an additional 5 minutes until the jackfruit is well coated and tender.
3. Spread the BBQ jackfruit mixture evenly over the pizza crust.
4. Top with red onion slices, bell peppers, and vegan cheese.

5. Bake in the preheated oven until the cheese has melted and the crust is crispy (follow the package instructions for baking time).
6. Remove from the oven, garnish with fresh cilantro, and let it cool slightly before slicing and serving.

Creole Cauliflower Pizza

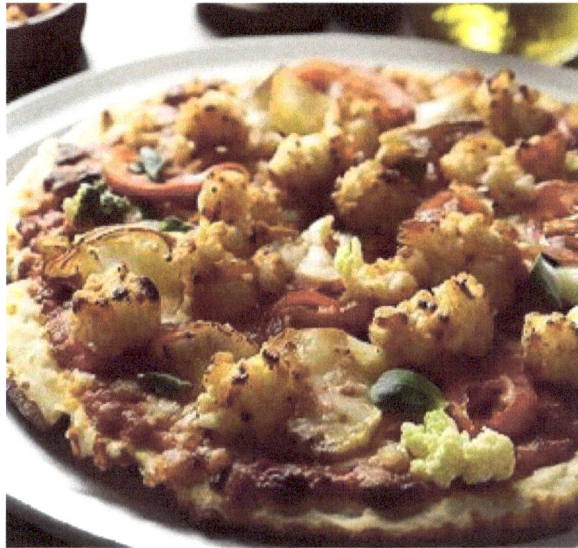

Prep Time: 20 minutes, Cook Time: 25 minutes, Servings: 4-6

Ingredients

- 1 vegan pre-made pizza crust
- 1 small head of cauliflower, cut into florets
- 1 tablespoon olive oil
- 2 teaspoons Creole seasoning
- 1/4 cup tomato sauce or marinara sauce
- 1/2 cup sliced vegan sausage or vegan pepperoni
- 1/2 green bell pepper, thinly sliced
- 1/2 red onion, thinly sliced
- 1 cup vegan cheese (such as vegan mozzarella or pepper jack)
- Fresh parsley, chopped (for garnish)

Instructions

1. Preheat the oven according to the pizza crust package instructions.
2. In a large bowl, toss the cauliflower florets with olive oil and Creole seasoning until well coated.

3. Spread the cauliflower evenly on a baking sheet and roast in the preheated oven for about 20 minutes until golden and tender.
4. Spread tomato sauce over the pizza crust.
5. Top with roasted cauliflower, vegan sausage or pepperoni, bell pepper slices, red onion slices, and vegan cheese.
6. Bake in the preheated oven according to the crust package instructions, until the cheese has melted and the crust is crispy.
7. Garnish with fresh parsley, slice, and serve.

Sweet Potato and Kale Pizza

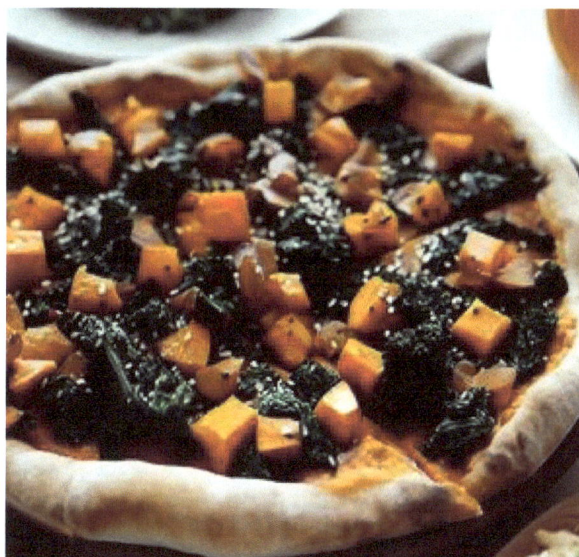

Prep Time: 20 minutes, Cook Time: 15 minutes, Servings: 4

Ingredients

- 1 vegan pre-made pizza crust
- 1 large sweet potato, peeled and thinly sliced
- 2 tablespoons olive oil, divided
- Salt and pepper to taste
- 1 cup chopped kale leaves
- 1/4 cup sliced red onion
- 1/2 cup vegan cheese (such as vegan mozzarella or goat cheese)
- 2 tablespoons balsamic glaze (optional)
- Fresh thyme leaves (for garnish)

Instructions

1. Preheat the oven according to the pizza crust package instructions.
2. In a bowl, toss the sweet potato slices with 1 tablespoon of olive oil, salt, and pepper.
3. Spread the sweet potato slices on a baking sheet and roast in the preheated oven for about 15 minutes until they are tender and slightly caramelized.

4. In a pan, heat the remaining tablespoon of olive oil and sauté the kale and red onion until the kale is wilted.
5. Spread the sautéed kale and onion mixture evenly over the pizza crust.
6. Top with roasted sweet potato slices and vegan cheese.
7. Bake in the preheated oven according to the crust package instructions, until the cheese has melted and the crust is crispy.
8. Drizzle with balsamic glaze (if desired) and garnish with fresh thyme leaves before serving.

Vegan Cornbread with a Soulful Twist

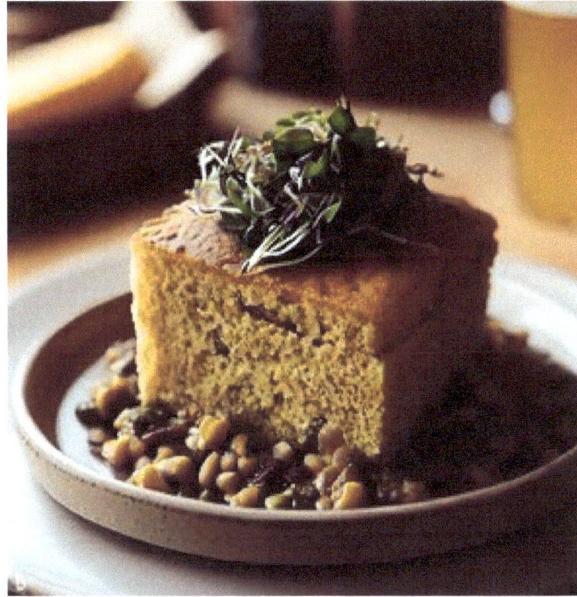

Prep Time: 10 minutes, Cook Time: 25-30 minutes, Servings: 8-10

Ingredients

- 1 cup cornmeal
- 1 cup all-purpose flour
- 1/4 cup coconut sugar
- 1 tablespoon baking powder
- 1/2 teaspoon baking soda
- 1/2 teaspoon salt
- 1 cup unsweetened almond milk (or any non-dairy milk of your choice)
- 1 tablespoon apple cider vinegar
- 1/4 cup melted coconut oil (or any other vegetable oil)
- 1/4 cup unsweetened applesauce
- 1/4 cup maple syrup
- 1/2 cup canned cream-style corn
- 1/4 cup chopped green onions
- 1/4 cup chopped red bell pepper
- 1/4 cup chopped fresh cilantro
- 1 jalapeño pepper, seeded and finely chopped (optional for a spicy kick)

Instructions

1. Preheat your oven to 375°F (190°C) and lightly grease a 9-inch square baking dish.
2. In a small bowl, combine the almond milk and apple cider vinegar. Set aside for a few minutes to curdle, creating a vegan "buttermilk."
3. In a large mixing bowl, whisk together the cornmeal, flour, coconut sugar, baking powder, baking soda, and salt.
4. In another bowl, combine the almond milk mixture, melted coconut oil, applesauce, and maple syrup. Whisk until well combined.
5. Pour the wet ingredients into the dry ingredients and stir until just combined.
6. Fold in the cream-style corn, green onions, red bell pepper, cilantro, and jalapeño pepper (if using). Mix gently until evenly distributed throughout the batter.
7. Pour the batter into the prepared baking dish and smooth the top with a spatula.
8. Bake in the preheated oven for 25-30 minutes or until the edges are golden brown and a toothpick inserted into the center comes out clean.
9. Remove from the oven and let it cool in the pan for 10 minutes.
10. Cut into squares and serve warm as a side dish or with your favorite soul food meal.

Classic Avocado Toast

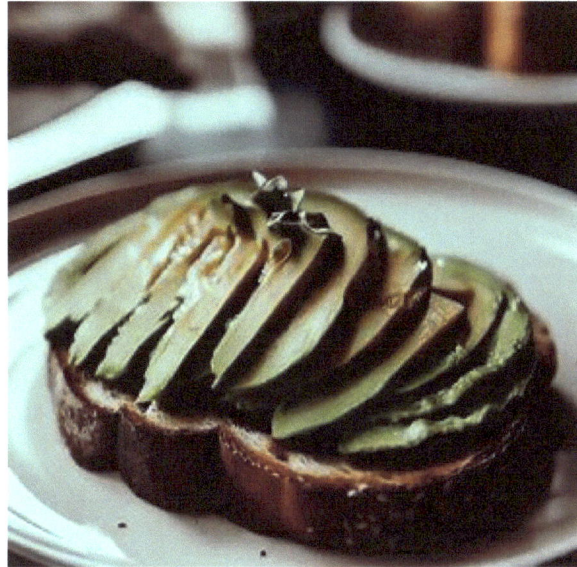

Prep Time: 5 minutes, Cook Time: 5 minutes, Servings: 2 servings

Ingredients

- 2 slices of whole-grain bread
- 1 ripe avocado
- Juice of 1/2 lemon
- Salt and pepper to taste
- Optional toppings: sliced cherry tomatoes, red pepper flakes, sprouts, or chopped cilantro

Instructions

1. Toast the bread slices until they're crispy.
2. Cut the avocado in half and remove the pit. Scoop out the flesh and place it in a bowl.
3. Mash the avocado with a fork and add lemon juice, salt, and pepper. Mix well.
4. Spread the mashed avocado mixture evenly onto the toasted bread slices.
5. Add your desired toppings such as sliced cherry tomatoes, red pepper flakes, sprouts, or chopped cilantro.
6. Serve immediately and enjoy!

Mediterranean Avocado Toast

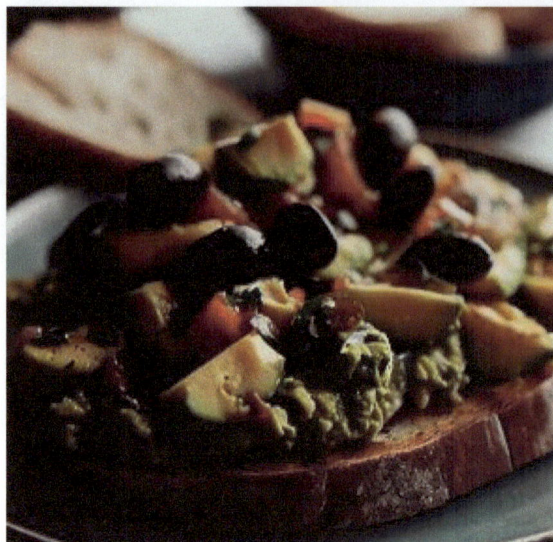

Prep Time: 10 minutes, Cook Time: 5 minutes, Servings: 2

Ingredients

- 2 slices of sourdough bread
- 1 ripe avocado
- 1 small cucumber, thinly sliced
- 2 tablespoons Kalamata olives, chopped 2 tablespoons sun-dried tomatoes, chopped 2 tablespoons fresh basil leaves, chopped
- Olive oil for drizzling
- Salt and pepper to taste

Instructions

1. Toast the sourdough bread slices until golden brown.
2. Cut the avocado in half, remove the pit, and scoop out the flesh into a bowl.
3. Mash the avocado with a fork and season with salt and pepper.
4. Spread the mashed avocado onto the toasted bread slices.
5. Top with cucumber slices, chopped Kalamata olives, sun-dried tomatoes, and fresh basil leaves.
6. Drizzle with olive oil and sprinkle with a little salt and pepper.
7. Serve immediately and enjoy!

Spicy Southwest Avocado Toast

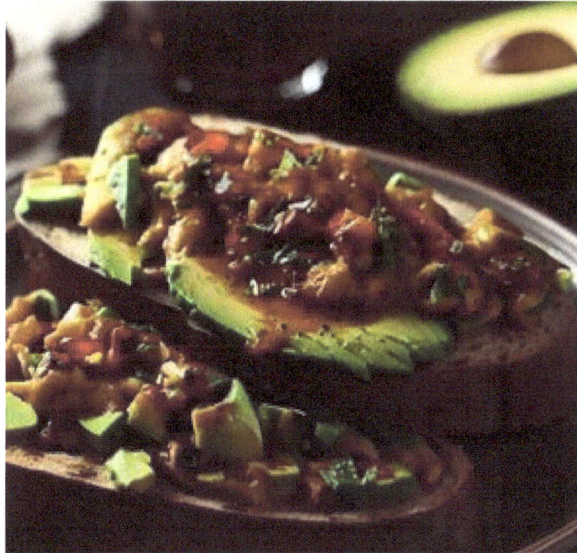

Prep Time: 10 minutes, Cook Time: 5 minutes, Servings: 2

Ingredients

- 2 slices of multigrain bread
- 1 ripe avocado
- 1/4 cup black beans, cooked and drained
- 1/4 cup corn kernels, cooked and drained
- 2 tablespoons red onion, finely chopped
- 2 tablespoons fresh cilantro, chopped
- 1/2 teaspoon cumin powder
- 1/4 teaspoon chili powder
- Juice of 1/2 lime
- Salt and pepper to taste

Instructions

1. Toast the multigrain bread slices until crispy.
2. Cut the avocado in half, remove the pit, and scoop out the flesh into a bowl.
3. Mash the avocado with a fork and add lime juice, cumin powder, chili powder, salt, and pepper. Mix well.

4. Spread the mashed avocado mixture onto the toasted bread slices.
5. Top with black beans, corn kernels, chopped red onion, and fresh cilantro.
6. Serve immediately and enjoy!

Quinoa Salad

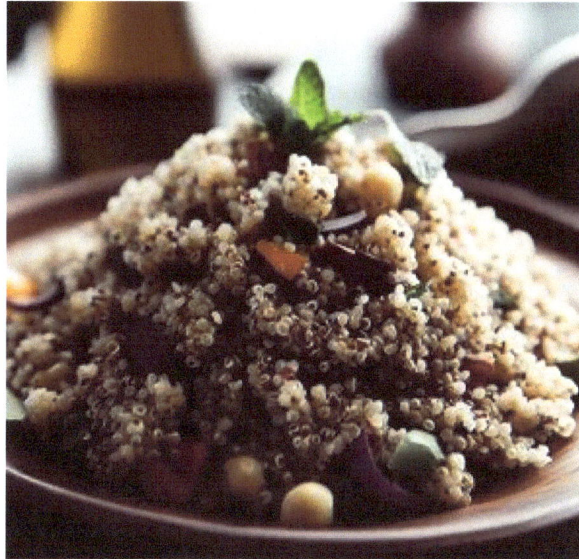

Prep Time: 15 minutes, Cook Time: 20 minutes, Servings: 4

Ingredients

- 1 cup quinoa, rinsed
- 2 cups water
- 1 cup cherry tomatoes, halved
- 1 cucumber, diced
- 1 bell pepper, diced
- 1/4 cup red onion, finely chopped
- 1/4 cup fresh parsley, chopped
- 1/4 cup fresh mint, chopped
- Juice of 1 lemon
- 2 tablespoons olive oil
- Salt and pepper to taste

Instructions

1. In a medium saucepan, bring the water to a boil.
2. Add the quinoa, reduce the heat to low, cover, and simmer for about 15-20 minutes, or until the water is absorbed and the quinoa is fluffy.

3. Remove the cooked quinoa from the heat and let it cool.
4. In a large bowl, combine the cherry tomatoes, cucumber, bell pepper, red onion, parsley, and mint.
5. In a small bowl, whisk together the lemon juice, olive oil, salt, and pepper.
6. Add the cooked quinoa to the bowl with the vegetables and pour the dressing over the salad.
7. Toss well to combine all the ingredients.
8. Adjust the seasoning if needed.
9. Serve the vegan quinoa salad chilled or at room temperature.

Coconut Curry Stir-Fry

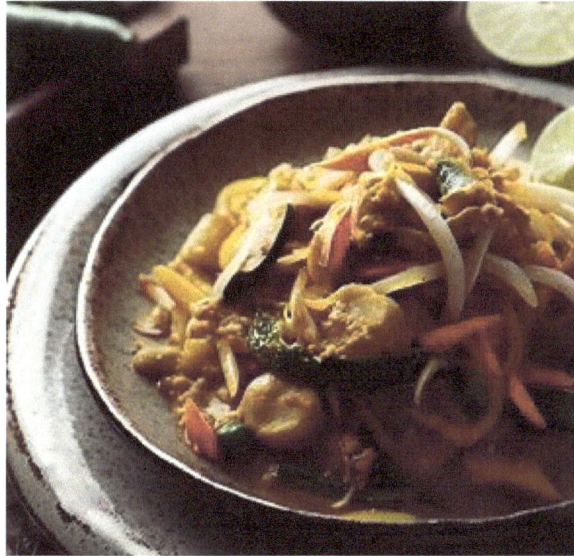

Prep Time: 15 minutes, Cook Time: 15 minutes, Servings: 4

Ingredients

- 1 tablespoon coconut oil
- 1 onion, sliced
- cloves garlic, minced
- 1 red pepper, sliced
- carrots, sliced
- 1 cup broccoli florets
- 1 cup snow peas
- 1 cup sliced mushrooms
- 1 can (14 oz) coconut milk
- 2 tablespoons red curry paste
- 2 tablespoons soy sauce or tamari sauce
- 1 tablespoon maple syrup
- Juice of 1 lime
- Fresh cilantro for garnish (optional)
- Cooked rice or noodles for serving

Instructions

1. Heat coconut oil in a large skillet or wok over medium heat.
2. Add the onion and garlic to the skillet and sauté until the onion becomes translucent.
3. Add the red pepper, carrots, broccoli, snow peas, and mushrooms to the skillet. Stir-fry for about 5-7 minutes until the vegetables are tender-crisp.
4. In a small bowl, whisk together the coconut milk, red curry paste, soy sauce or tamari sauce, maple syrup, and lime juice.
5. Pour the curry sauce over the vegetables in the skillet and stir well to combine.
6. Continue to cook for another 3-5 minutes until the sauce is heated through.
7. Garnish with fresh cilantro, if desired.
8. Serve the vegan coconut curry stir-fry over cooked rice or noodles.

Chickpea Salad Sandwich

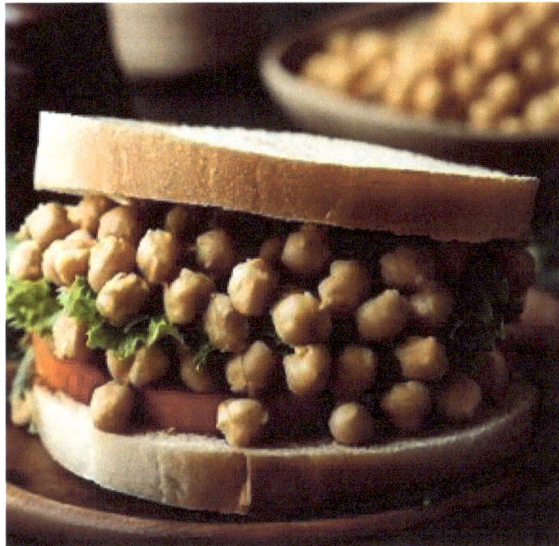

Prep Time: 10 minutes, Servings: 4

Ingredients

- 1 can (14 oz) chickpeas, drained and rinsed
- 1/4 cup vegan mayonnaise
- 1 tablespoon Dijon mustard
- 2 stalks celery, diced
- 1/4 cup red onion, diced
- 2 tablespoons fresh dill, chopped
- Salt and pepper to taste
- Bread or rolls for serving
- Lettuce and tomato slices for topping

Instructions

1. In a mixing bowl, mash the chickpeas with a fork or potato masher until chunky.
2. Add the vegan mayonnaise, Dijon mustard, celery, red onion, and fresh dill to the bowl. Stir well to combine.
3. Season with salt and pepper to taste.
4. Spread the chickpea salad mixture onto bread or rolls.
5. Top with lettuce and tomato slices.
6. Serve the vegan chickpea salad sandwiches.

Stuffed Bell Peppers

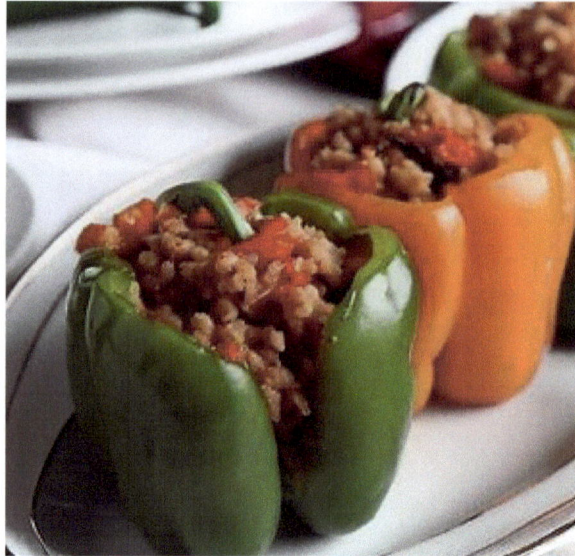

Prep Time: 15 minutes, Cook Time: 45 minutes, Servings: 4

Ingredients

- 4 bell peppers, any color
- 1 tablespoon olive oil
- 1 onion, diced
- 3 cloves garlic, minced
- 1 zucchini, diced
- 1 cup cooked quinoa
- 1 can (14 oz) diced tomatoes
- 1 teaspoon dried basil
- 1 teaspoon dried oregano
- Salt and pepper to taste
- Vegan cheese, shredded (optional)

Instructions

1. Preheat the oven to 375°F (190°C).
2. Slice the tops off the bell peppers and remove the seeds and membranes.
3. In a large skillet, heat the olive oil over medium heat.

4. Add the onion, garlic, and zucchini to the skillet. Sauté until the vegetables start to soften.
5. Stir in the cooked quinoa, diced tomatoes (with their juice), dried basil, dried oregano, salt, and pepper.
6. Cook for another 5 minutes, allowing the flavors to combine.
7. Spoon the quinoa mixture into the bell peppers, filling them evenly.
8. Place the stuffed bell peppers in a baking dish and cover with foil.
9. Bake in the preheated oven for 35 minutes.
10. If desired, remove the foil and sprinkle vegan cheese on top of each bell pepper.
11. Return to the oven and bake for another 10 minutes, or until the bell peppers are tender and the cheese is melted.
12. Serve the vegan stuffed bell peppers hot.

Snacks and Desserts

Chocolate Chip Cookies

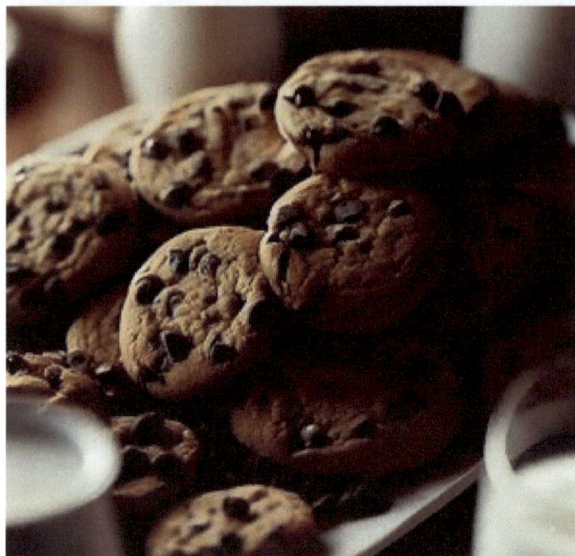

Prep Time: 15 minutes, Cook Time: 10 minutes, Servings: 24 cookies

Ingredients

- 1/2 cup vegan butter, softened
- 3/4 cup palm sugar
- 1/4 cup coconut sugar
- 1/4 cup unsweetened applesauce
- 1 teaspoon vanilla extract
- 2 cups all-purpose flour
- 1 teaspoon baking soda
- 1/2 teaspoon salt
- 1 cup vegan chocolate chips

Instructions

1. Preheat the oven to 350°F (175°C). Line a baking sheet with parchment paper.
2. In a large mixing bowl, cream together the vegan butter, palm sugar, and coconut sugar until light and fluffy.
3. Add the applesauce and vanilla extract to the bowl and mix until well combined.
4. In a separate bowl, whisk together the flour, baking soda, and salt.
5. Gradually add the dry ingredients to the wet ingredients, mixing until just combined.
6. Fold in the vegan chocolate chips.
7. Drop rounded tablespoons of dough onto the prepared baking sheet, spacing them about 2 inches apart.
8. Bake for 10-12 minutes, or until the edges are golden brown.
9. Remove from the oven and let cool on the baking sheet for a few minutes before transferring to a wire rack to cool completely.

Black Bean Brownies

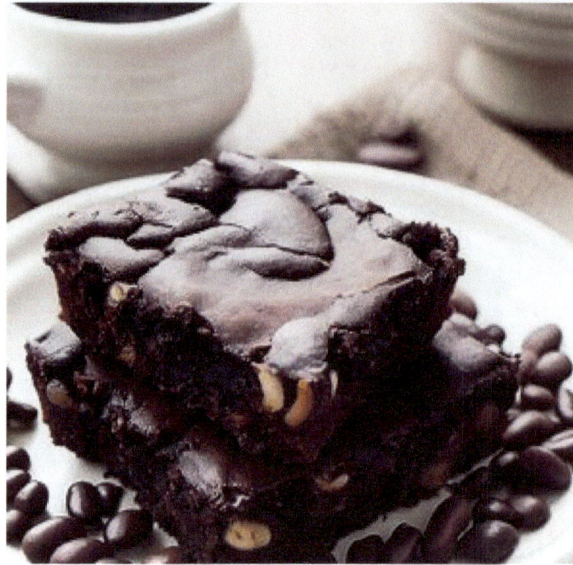

Prep Time: 15 minutes, Cook Time: 25 minutes, Servings: 9

Ingredients

- 1 can (15 oz) black beans, drained and rinsed
- 1/2 cup cocoa powder
- 1/2 cup maple syrup
- 1/4 cup almond butter
- 1/4 cup oat flour
- 1/4 cup non-dairy milk
- 2 teaspoons vanilla extract
- 1/2 teaspoon baking powder
- 1/4 teaspoon salt
- 1/2 cup vegan chocolate chips (optional)

Instructions

1. Preheat the oven to 350°F (175°C). Grease or line an 8x8-inch baking pan.
2. In a food processor, combine the black beans, cocoa powder, maple syrup, almond butter, oat flour, non-dairy milk, vanilla

extract, baking powder, and salt. Blend until smooth and well combined.

3. Stir in the chocolate chips, if using.

4. Pour the batter into the prepared baking pan and spread it evenly.

5. Bake for 25 minutes, or until a toothpick inserted into the center comes out with a few crumbs.

6. Remove from the oven and let cool completely before cutting into squares.

Banana Bread

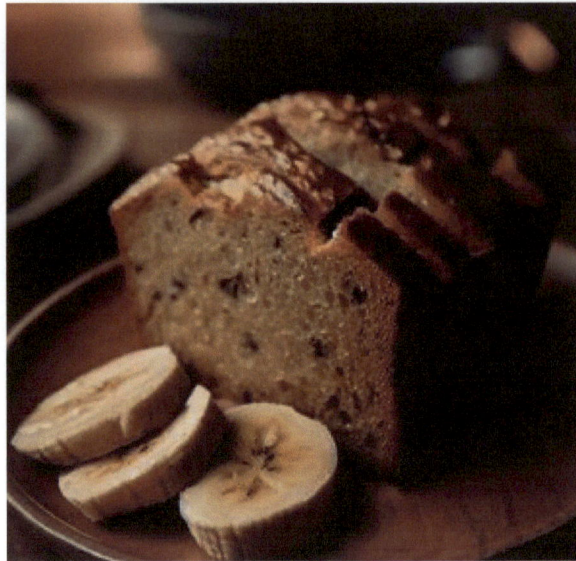

Prep Time: 10 minutes, Cook Time: 50-60 minutes, Servings: 8

Ingredients

- 3 ripe bananas, mashed
- 1/2 cup maple syrup
- 1/4 cup plant-based milk
- 1 teaspoon vanilla extract
- 2 cups all-purpose flour
- 1 teaspoon baking soda
- 1/2 teaspoon salt
- 1/2 teaspoon cinnamon
- 1/4 cup melted coconut oil
- 1/2 cup chopped walnuts (optional)

Instructions

1. Preheat the oven to 350°F (175°C) and grease a loaf pan.
2. In a large mixing bowl, combine mashed bananas, maple syrup, plant-based milk, and vanilla extract.
3. In a separate bowl, whisk together the flour, baking soda, salt, and cinnamon.

4. Gradually add the dry ingredients to the wet ingredients, mixing until just combined.
5. Stir in the melted coconut oil and chopped walnuts, if using.
6. Pour the batter into the prepared loaf pan and smooth the top.
7. Bake for 50-60 minutes, or until a toothpick inserted into the center comes out clean.
8. Allow the banana bread to cool in the pan for 10 minutes, then transfer it to a wire rack to cool completely.
9. Slice and serve the vegan banana bread as a delicious breakfast or snack.

Corn Bread

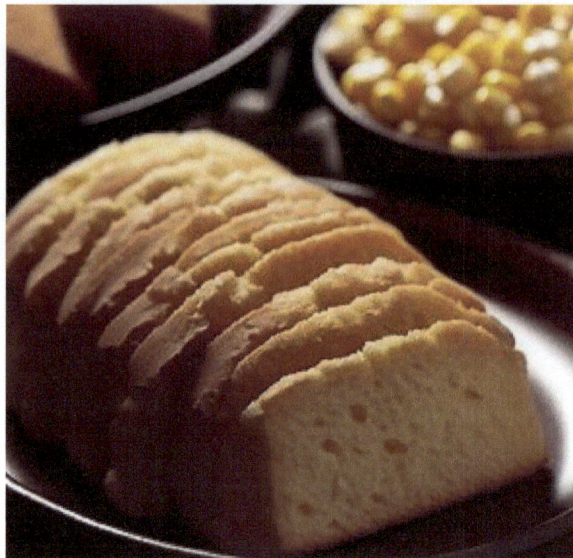

Prep Time: 10 minutes, Cook Time: 25 minutes, Servings: 8

Ingredients

- 1 cup cornmeal
- 1 cup all-purpose flour
- 1/4 cup palm sugar
- 1 tablespoon baking powder
- 1/2 teaspoon salt
- 1 cup unsweetened almond milk (or any non-dairy milk)
- 1/4 cup melted vegan butter
- 1/4 cup unsweetened applesauce
- 1 cup corn kernels (fresh or frozen)

Instructions

1. Preheat your oven to 400°F (200°C). Grease a 9-inch square baking pan and set aside.
2. In a large mixing bowl, combine the cornmeal, flour, palm sugar, baking powder, and salt.
3. In a separate bowl, whisk together the almond milk, melted vegan butter, and applesauce until well combined.

4. Pour the wet ingredients into the dry ingredients and mix until just combined. Do not overmix.
5. Gently fold in the corn kernels.
6. Pour the batter into the prepared baking pan and spread it evenly.
7. Bake in the preheated oven for about 20-25 minutes or until a toothpick inserted into the center comes out clean.
8. Remove from the oven and let it cool for a few minutes before cutting into squares.
9. Serve warm and enjoy!

Blueberry Muffins

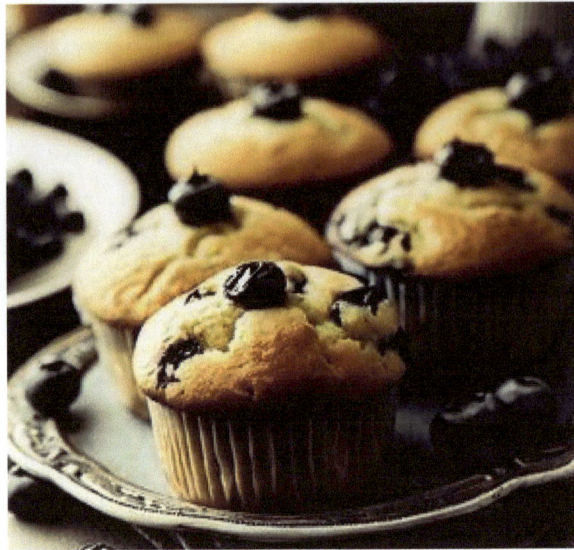

Prep Time: 15 minutes, Cook Time: 20-25 minutes, Servings: 12 muffins

Ingredients

- 2 cups all-purpose flour
- 1/2 cup palm sugar
- 1 tablespoon baking powder
- 1/2 teaspoon baking soda
- 1/4 teaspoon salt
- 1 cup plant-based milk
- 1/4 cup coconut oil, melted
- 1/4 cup applesauce
- 1 teaspoon vanilla extract
- 1 cup fresh blueberries

Instructions

1. Preheat the oven to 375°F (190°C) and line a muffin tin with paper liners.
2. In a large mixing bowl, whisk together the flour, palm sugar, baking powder, baking soda, and salt.

3. In a separate bowl, combine the plant-based milk, melted coconut oil, applesauce, and vanilla extract.
4. Pour the wet ingredients into the dry ingredients and mix until just combined.
5. Gently fold in the fresh blueberries.
6. Divide the batter evenly among the prepared muffin cups, filling each about 2/3 full.
7. Bake for 20-25 minutes, or until a toothpick inserted into the center of a muffin comes out clean.
8. Remove the muffins from the oven and let them cool in the tin for 5 minutes, then transfer them to a wire rack to cool completely.

Peach Cobbler

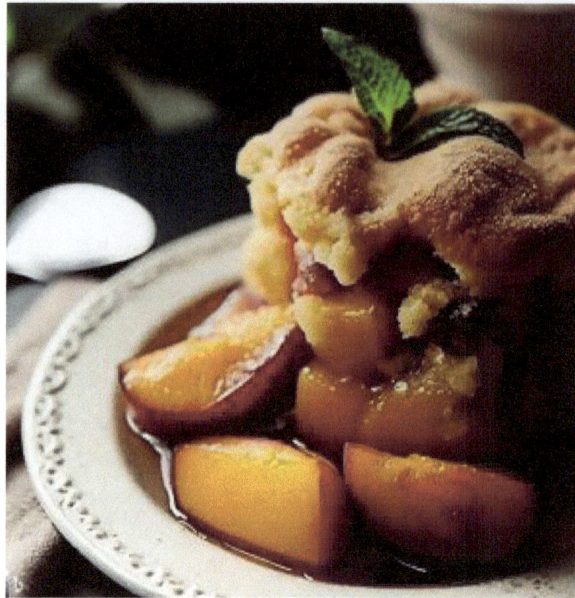

Prep Time: 20 minutes, Cook Time: 50 minutes, Servings: 6-8

Enjoy the soulful vegan peach cobbler, with its sweet and juicy filling and tender cornmeal cobbler topping!

For the Peach Filling:

- 6 cups sliced peaches (fresh or frozen)
- 1/2 cup palm sugar
- 1 tablespoon lemon juice
- 1 teaspoon vanilla extract
- 1/2 teaspoon ground cinnamon
- 1/4 teaspoon ground nutmeg

For the Cobbler Topping:

- 1 1/2 cups all-purpose flour
- 1/2 cup cornmeal
- 1/2 cup palm sugar
- 2 teaspoons baking powder
- 1/2 teaspoon salt
- 1/2 cup vegan butter, melted
- 1 cup plant-based milk (such as almond or soy milk)

- 1 teaspoon vanilla extract

For Serving:

- Vegan vanilla ice cream or whipped cream (optional)

Instructions

1. Preheat your oven to 375°F (190°C). Grease a 9x13-inch baking dish or a similar-sized oven-safe dish.
2. In a large bowl, combine the sliced peaches, granulated sugar, lemon juice, vanilla extract, ground cinnamon, and ground nutmeg. Toss to coat the peaches evenly in the mixture.
3. Pour the peach filling into the greased baking dish and spread it out in an even layer.
4. In a separate bowl, whisk together the all-purpose flour, cornmeal, granulated sugar, baking powder, and salt for the cobbler topping.
5. Add the melted vegan butter, plant-based milk, and vanilla extract to the dry ingredients. Stir until just combined, being careful not to overmix.
6. Drop spoonful of the cobbler topping evenly over the peach filling, covering as much of the surface as possible.
7. Bake the peach cobbler in the preheated oven for 40-45 minutes, or until the filling is bubbly and the cobbler topping is golden brown.
8. Remove from the oven and let it cool for a few minutes before serving.
9. Serve the warm vegan peach cobbler as is or with a scoop of vegan vanilla ice cream or whipped cream for an extra special touch.

Granola Bars

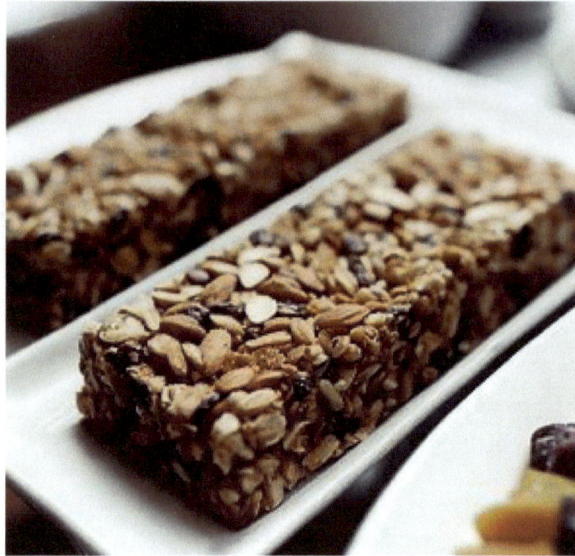

Prep Time: 15 minutes, Cook Time: 20 minutes, Servings: 12 bars

Ingredients

- 1 1/2 cups rolled oats
- 1 cup puffed rice cereal
- 1/2 cup almonds, chopped
- 1/4 cup unsweetened shredded coconut
- 1/4 cup almond butter
- 1/4 cup maple syrup
- 1/4 cup coconut oil, melted
- 1 teaspoon vanilla extract
- 1/4 teaspoon salt
- 1/2 cup dried fruit (e.g., cranberries, raisins, chopped dates)

Instructions

1. Preheat the oven to 350°F (175°C). Line an 8x8-inch baking dish with parchment paper.
2. In a large mixing bowl, combine the rolled oats, puffed rice cereal, chopped almonds, and shredded coconut.

3. In a separate bowl, whisk together the almond butter, maple syrup, melted coconut oil, vanilla extract, and salt until well combined.
4. Pour the wet ingredients over the dry ingredients and mix until evenly coated.
5. Fold in the dried fruit.
6. Transfer the mixture to the prepared baking dish and press it down firmly using a spatula or the back of a spoon.
7. Bake for 18-20 minutes, or until the edges are golden brown.
8. Remove from the oven and let cool completely in the dish before cutting into bars.

Sweet Potato Fries

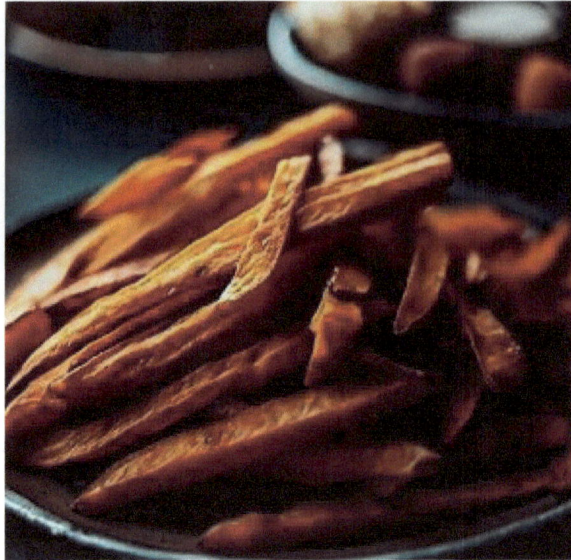

Prep Time: 10 minutes, Cook Time: 25 minutes, Servings: 4

Ingredients

- 2 large sweet potatoes
- 2 tablespoons olive oil
- 1 teaspoon paprika
- 1/2 teaspoon garlic powder
- 1/2 teaspoon salt
- 1/4 teaspoon black pepper

Instructions

1. Preheat the oven to 425°F (220°C). Line a baking sheet with parchment paper.
2. Wash and peel the sweet potatoes. Cut them into thin, even-sized fries.
3. In a large bowl, toss the sweet potato fries with olive oil, paprika, garlic powder, salt, and black pepper until well coated.
4. Arrange the fries in a single layer on the prepared baking sheet.
5. Bake for 20-25 minutes, flipping once halfway through, until the fries are crispy and golden brown.
6. Remove from the oven and let cool slightly before serving.

Okra Fries

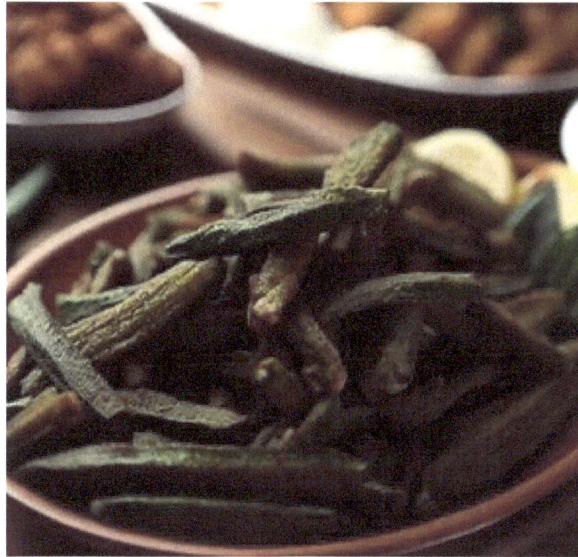

Prep Time: 15 minutes, Cook Time: 20 minutes, Servings: 4

Ingredients

- 1-pound fresh okra
- 1/2 cup all-purpose flour
- 1/4 cup cornmeal
- 1 teaspoon garlic powder
- 1 teaspoon paprika
- 1/2 teaspoon salt
- 1/4 teaspoon black pepper
- 2 large eggs, beaten
- Cooking oil, for frying

Instructions

1. Wash the okra thoroughly and trim off the tops and tips. Slice the okra pods lengthwise into thin strips, resembling French fries.
2. In a shallow dish, combine the flour, cornmeal, garlic powder, paprika, salt, and black pepper. Mix well.
3. Dip the okra slices into the beaten eggs, allowing any excess to drip off, and then coat them in the flour mixture. Make sure each slice is evenly coated.

4. In a large skillet, heat enough cooking oil to cover the bottom of the pan over medium-high heat.
5. Once the oil is hot, carefully place the coated okra slices in a single layer in the skillet. Cook them in batches if necessary, ensuring not to overcrowd the pan.
6. Fry the okra slices for about 2-3 minutes on each side, or until they turn golden brown and crispy. Use tongs or a slotted spoon to flip them halfway through cooking.
7. Once the okra fries are cooked, transfer them to a paper towel-lined plate to drain any excess oil.
8. Repeat the frying process with the remaining okra slices until they are all cooked.
9. Serve the Okra Fries immediately while still hot. They can be enjoyed as a snack or a side dish with your favorite dipping sauce.

Hummus

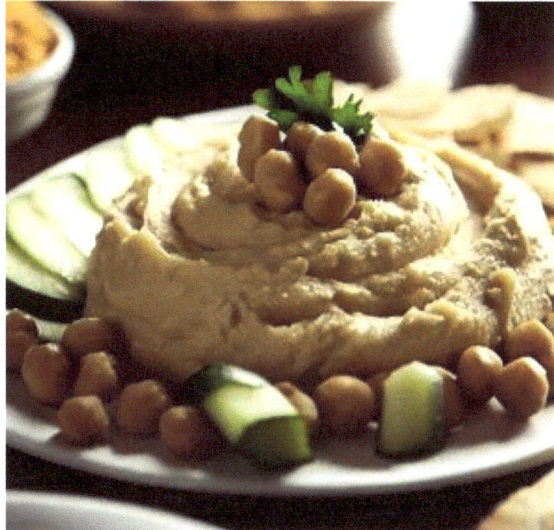

Prep Time: 10 minutes, Servings: 8

Ingredients

- 1 can (15 oz) chickpeas, drained and rinsed
- 1/4 cup tahini
- 2 tablespoons lemon juice
- 2 tablespoons olive oil
- 1 clove garlic, minced
- 1/2 teaspoon cumin
- 1/2 teaspoon salt
- Water (as needed)

Instructions

1. Place the chickpeas, tahini, lemon juice, olive oil, garlic, cumin, and salt in a food processor or blender.
2. Process until smooth and creamy. If the hummus is too thick, add water, a tablespoon at a time, until desired consistency is reached.
3. Taste and adjust the seasoning if needed.
4. Transfer the hummus to a serving bowl and drizzle with olive oil, if desired.
5. Serve with pita bread, fresh vegetables, or your favorite crackers.

Plantain Chips

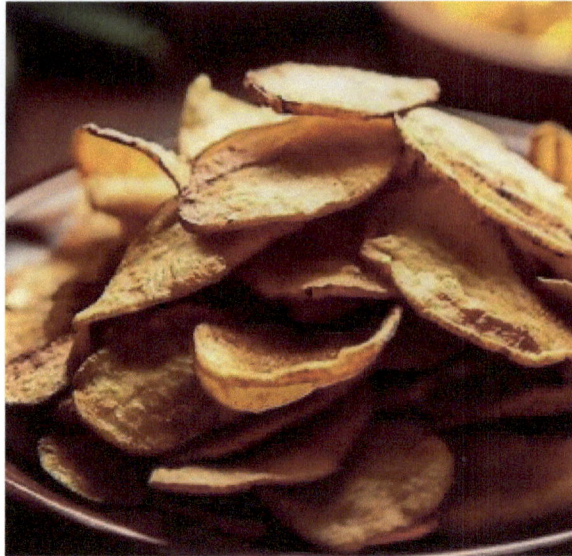

Prep Time: 10 minutes, Cook Time: 20 minutes, Servings: 4

Ingredients

- 2 ripe plantains
- 2 tablespoons olive oil
- 1/2 teaspoon paprika
- 1/2 teaspoon garlic powder
- 1/4 teaspoon salt

Instructions

1. Preheat the oven to 400°F (200°C). Line a baking sheet with parchment paper.
2. Peel the plantains and cut them into thin slices.
3. In a bowl, toss the plantain slices with olive oil, paprika, garlic powder, and salt until well coated.
4. Arrange the plantain slices in a single layer on the prepared baking sheet.
5. Bake for 15-20 minutes, flipping once halfway through, until the chips are crispy and lightly golden.
6. Remove from the oven and let cool before serving.

Energy Balls

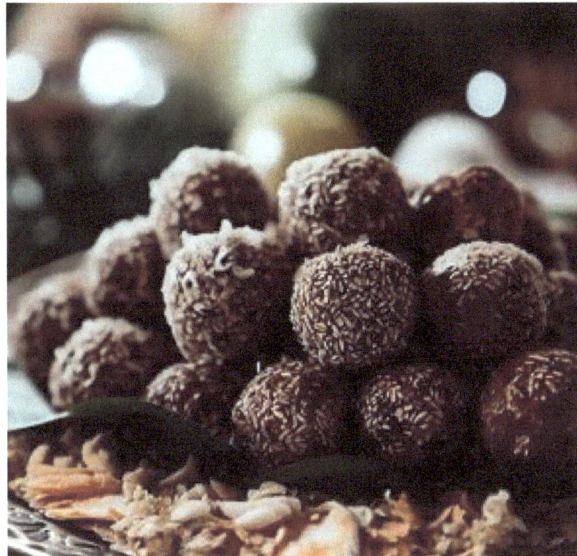

Prep Time: 10 minutes, Servings: 12

Ingredients

- 1 cup pitted dates
- 1/2 cup almonds
- 1/2 cup rolled oats
- 2 tablespoons cocoa powder
- 2 tablespoons almond butter
- 1 tablespoon maple syrup
- 1/2 teaspoon vanilla extract
- Pinch of salt
- Desiccated coconut, for rolling (optional)

Instructions

1. Place the dates, almonds, rolled oats, cocoa powder, almond butter, maple syrup, vanilla extract, and salt in a food processor. Blend until the mixture comes together and forms a sticky dough.
2. Scoop out about a tablespoon of the dough and roll it into a ball using your hands. Repeat with the remaining dough.

3. If desired, roll the energy balls in desiccated coconut for added texture and flavor.
4. Place the energy balls in an airtight container and refrigerate for at least 30 minutes to firm up.
5. Serve chilled and enjoy as a quick and energizing snack.

Chia Seed Pudding

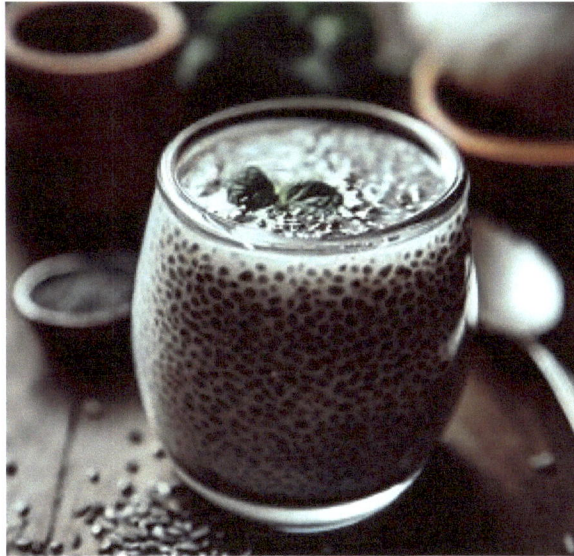

Prep Time: 5 minutes (plus overnight chilling), Cook Time: 0 minutes, Servings: 2

Ingredients

- 1/4 cup chia seeds
- 1 cup milk (dairy or plant-based)
- 1-2 tablespoons honey or maple syrup, to taste
- 1/2 teaspoon vanilla extract
- Optional toppings: fresh fruits, nuts, coconut flakes, cinnamon, etc.

Instructions

1. In a bowl or jar, combine the chia seeds, milk, honey or maple syrup, and vanilla extract. Stir well to ensure the chia seeds are evenly distributed.
2. Let the mixture sit for a few minutes, then stir again to prevent clumping of the chia seeds.
3. Cover the bowl or jar and refrigerate it overnight or for at least 4-6 hours, allowing the chia seeds to absorb the liquid and thicken into a pudding-like consistency.

4. After chilling, give the chia seed pudding a good stir to break up any clumps that may have formed. If the pudding is too thick, you can add a little more milk to achieve the desired consistency.
5. Taste the chia seed pudding and adjust the sweetness if needed by adding more honey or maple syrup.
6. Divide the chia seed pudding into serving bowls or glasses.
7. If desired, add your favorite toppings such as fresh fruits, nuts, coconut flakes, or a sprinkle of cinnamon.
8. Serve the Chia Seed Pudding immediately or return it to the refrigerator until ready to serve.

Banana Nice Cream

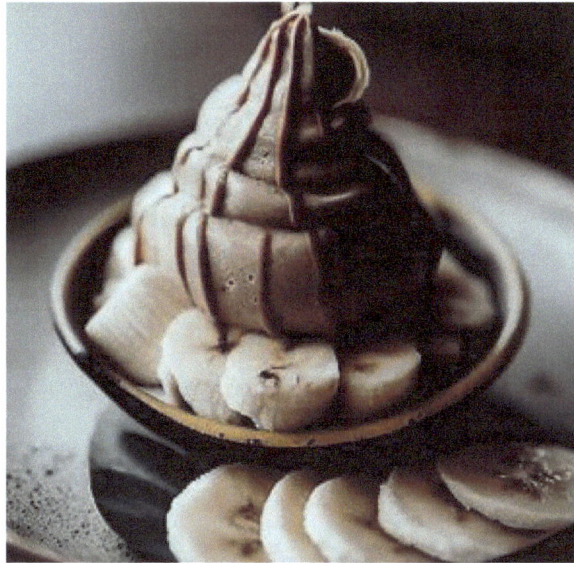

Prep Time: 5 minutes, Servings: 2

Ingredients

- 2 ripe bananas, peeled and sliced
- 2 tablespoons almond butter
- 1 tablespoon maple syrup
- 1/2 teaspoon vanilla extract
- Optional toppings: chopped nuts, shredded coconut, chocolate chips, fresh fruit

Instructions

1. Place the sliced bananas in a Ziploc bag and freeze for at least 4 hours or overnight.
2. In a blender or food processor, combine the frozen banana slices, almond butter, maple syrup, and vanilla extract.
3. Blend until smooth and creamy, scraping down the sides as needed.
4. Transfer the nice cream to bowls and add your favorite toppings.
5. Serve immediately and enjoy a refreshing and guilt-free dessert.

Peanut Butter Banana Ice Cream

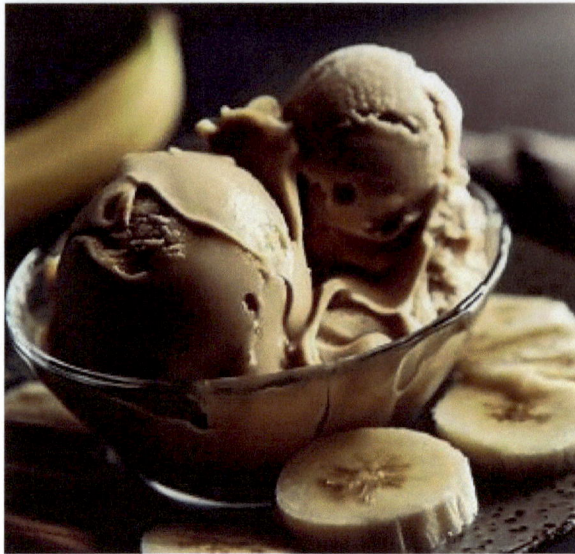

Prep Time: 5 minutes, Cook Time: 0 minutes (freezing time required),
Servings: 4

Ingredients

- 4 ripe bananas, peeled and sliced
- 1/2 cup creamy peanut butter
- 1/4 cup honey or maple syrup (optional for added sweetness)
- 1 teaspoon vanilla extract
- Optional toppings: chopped peanuts, chocolate chips, caramel sauce, sliced bananas, etc.

Instructions

1. Place the sliced bananas in a single layer on a baking sheet lined with parchment paper. Freeze the banana slices for at least 2-3 hours or until solid.
2. Once the banana slices are frozen, transfer them to a food processor or high-powered blender.
3. Add the creamy peanut butter, honey or maple syrup (if using), and vanilla extract to the food processor or blender.

4. Blend the mixture on high speed until the ingredients are well combined and the mixture becomes smooth and creamy. You may need to stop and scrape down the sides of the container a few times during blending.
5. Taste the mixture and adjust the sweetness if desired by adding more honey or maple syrup.
6. Once the mixture is smooth and creamy, transfer it to an airtight container and place it in the freezer for about 1-2 hours to firm up slightly.
7. After the ice cream has firmed up, it's ready to serve. Scoop the Peanut Butter Banana Ice Cream into bowls or cones.
8. If desired, garnish with your favorite toppings such as chopped peanuts, chocolate chips, caramel sauce, or sliced bananas.
9. Serve immediately and enjoy your homemade Peanut Butter Banana Ice Cream!

Watermelon Mint Popsicles

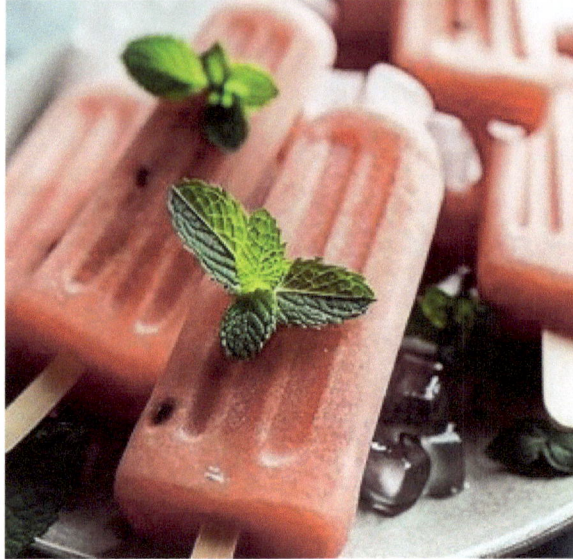

Prep Time: 10 minutes, Cook Time: 0 minutes (freezing time required),
Servings: 6 popsicles

Ingredients

- 4 cups seedless watermelon, diced
- 1 tablespoon fresh mint leaves, chopped
- 1 tablespoon fresh lime juice
- Optional: 1-2 tablespoons honey or sweetener of your choice, to taste

Instructions

1. Place the diced watermelon in a blender or food processor. Blend until smooth and no chunks remain.
2. Add the chopped mint leaves and lime juice to the blender or food processor. Blend again until the mint is well incorporated into the watermelon mixture.
3. Taste the mixture and add honey or any preferred sweetener if desired. Blend briefly to combine.
4. Pour the watermelon mixture into popsicle molds, leaving a small gap at the top to allow for expansion during freezing.

5. If using popsicle molds with sticks, insert the sticks into the molds. If using molds without sticks, cover the molds with their respective lids or use aluminum foil with slits to hold the sticks in place.
6. Place the popsicle molds in the freezer and let them freeze for at least 4-6 hours, or until completely solid.
7. Once the watermelon popsicles are frozen, remove them from the molds by running warm water over the bottom of the molds. Gently pull the popsicles out.
8. Serve the Watermelon Mint Popsicles immediately and enjoy the refreshing treat on a hot day!

CHAPTER FOURTEEN

The Importance of Community and Support

- Building a supportive network
- Engaging with vegan communities online and offline
- Celebrating cultural diversity within the vegan movement
- Sharing success stories and inspiring others

Surrounding oneself with a supportive network is essential when adopting a vegan lifestyle. It not only makes the transition easier but also enhances the overall experience. In this chapter, we will delve into various strategies to cultivate a strong support system that fosters encouragement, offers valuable resources, and facilitates shared experiences.

One effective approach to building a supportive network is by connecting with like-minded individuals. The vegan community is vast and diverse, encompassing people from different walks of life. By finding individuals who share your passion for veganism, you can create a sense of camaraderie and understanding. Online platforms and social media are excellent resources for connecting with the vegan community, as they provide spaces for discussions, sharing ideas, and seeking advice. Engaging with online communities not only allows you to connect with individuals from around the world but also provides access to valuable information, recipes, and resources.

However, while online engagement is beneficial, it's equally important to foster offline interactions. Attending local vegan events or joining community organizations can provide opportunities to meet fellow vegans in person, forge deeper connections, and build lasting friendships. These offline interactions offer a chance to engage in meaningful conversations, exchange personal stories, and learn from others' experiences. By participating in local vegan events, you can immerse yourself in the vibrant vegan culture of your community and discover new ideas and perspectives.

Furthermore, it's crucial to acknowledge and celebrate the cultural diversity within the vegan movement. Veganism is not limited to any particular culture or background; it transcends borders and unites individuals from all walks of life. Embracing different culinary traditions and exploring the rich tapestry of plant-based cuisine from various cultures can be an exciting and rewarding aspect of the vegan lifestyle. By sharing and celebrating these diverse culinary experiences, we can inspire others to adopt veganism and appreciate the multitude of flavors and dishes available.

Lastly, this chapter encourages readers to share their own stories, recipes, and insights. By contributing your experiences and successes, you can inspire and motivate others who may be on their own journey toward a vegan lifestyle. Your unique perspective can create a ripple effect of positive change, as your stories resonate with others and empower them to make compassionate choices.

In summary, creating a supportive network is crucial for a successful and enjoyable vegan journey. By connecting with like-minded individuals both online and offline, embracing cultural diversity, and sharing personal experiences, we can cultivate a thriving community that uplifts and inspires one another.

CHAPTER FIFTEEN

Conclusion

- Recap of key points discussed in the e-book
- Encouragement for readers to take steps toward a healthier lifestyle
- Final thoughts on the transformative power of Veganism

This final chapter summarizes the key points covered throughout the book, emphasizing the importance of understanding the impact of diets on health, particularly within the challenges faced by the Black community. It also highlights the potential benefits of adopting a vegan lifestyle. By taking steps towards a healthier lifestyle, readers can positively change their dietary habits and improve their overall well-being. It's important to recognize that even small changes can have a significant impact on health. In addition to personal health, the book reflects on the transformative power of veganism for the environment and social justice. It encourages readers to embrace a compassionate and sustainable lifestyle that aligns with their values and promotes positive change in various aspects of life. By incorporating these principles into their lives, readers can make a difference not only for themselves but also for the wider community, fostering a healthier, more equitable, and environmentally conscious future.

REFERENCES AND RESOURCES

INTRODUCTION

Citations:

1. A. Satija, S. N. Bhupathiraju, E. B. Rimm, D. Spiegelman, S. E. Chiuve, L. Borgi, et al. (2016). Results from three prospective cohort studies on plant-based eating habits and the incidence of type 2 diabetes in men and women in the United States. Medical PLoS, 13(6), e1002039.
2. Nkonde, C., Chedid, R. A., & Golden, S. H. (2020). Food deserts: causes, consequences, and solutions. Current Diabetes Reports, 20(11), 1-8.
3. Hu, F. B. (2002). Dietary pattern analysis: a new direction in nutritional epidemiology. Current Opinion in Lipidology, 13(1), 3-9.
4. Satija, A., Bhupathiraju, S. N., Rimm, E. B., Spiegelman, D., Chiuve, S. E., Borgi, L., ... & Willett, W. (2016). Plant-based dietary patterns and incidence of type 2 diabetes in US men and women: results from three prospective cohort studies. PLoS Medicine, 13(6), e1002039.
5. Satia, J. A., & Galanko, J. A. (2007). Demographic, behavioral, psychosocial, and dietary correlates of cancer screening in African Americans. Preventive Medicine, 44(4), 312-320.
6. Craig, W. J., & Mangels, A. R. (2009). Position of the American Dietetic Association: vegetarian diets. Journal of the American Dietetic Association, 109(7), 1266-1282.

CHAPTER ONE

Citations:

1. "The Slave Community: Plantation Life in the Antebellum South" by John W. Blassingame - This influential work examines the social and cultural lives of enslaved African Americans, including aspects of their diet and food culture.
2. "Soul Food: The Surprising Story of an American Cuisine, One Plate at a Time" by Adrian Miller - This book explores the history and significance of soul food, tracing its roots to the food ways of enslaved Africans and the adaptations made during slavery and beyond.
3. "Food and the African American: A Journey to Soul" edited by Doris Witt - This anthology delves into the historical, cultural, and political dimensions of the African American diet, offering insights into the culinary legacy of African Americans.
4. "High on the Hog: A Culinary Journey from Africa to America" by Jessica B. Harris - In this book, Jessica B. Harris examines the connections between African and African American food traditions, highlighting the impact of slavery on the development of African American cuisine.
5. "The Jemima Code: Two Centuries of African American Cookbooks" by Toni Tipton-Martin - This book explores the history of African American cookbooks, providing valuable insights into the culinary traditions and contributions of African Americans throughout history

Articles:

- Bower, A. B. (2017). The African American Experience: An Historiographical and Bibliographical Guide. ABC-CLIO.
- Blassingame, J. W. (1979). The Slave Community: Plantation Life in the Antebellum South. Oxford University Press.
- Fett, S. (2002). Working Cures: Healing, Health, and Power on Southern Slave Plantations. University of North Carolina Press.
- Opie, F. G. (2008). Hog and Hominy: Soul Food from Africa to America. Columbia University Press.
- Painter, N. I. (2007). Soul Food: The Surprising Story of an American Cuisine, One Plate at a Time. University of North Carolina Press.
- Twitty, M. W. (2017). The Cooking Gene: A Journey Through African American Culinary History in the Old South. Amistad.
- White, D. G. (2011). The Ideology of Slavery: Proslavery Thought in the Antebellum South, 1830-1860. Louisiana State University Press.
- Willis, L. M. (2019). Building Houses Out of Chicken Legs: Black Women, Food, and Power. University of North Carolina Press.

CHAPTER TWO

Citations:

1. Appel, L. J., Moore, T. J., Obarzanek, E., Vollmer, W. M., Svetkey, L. P., Sacks, F. M.,... & Kennedy, B. M. (1997). A clinical trial of the effects of dietary patterns on blood pressure. New England Journal of Medicine, 336(16), 1117-1124.
2. Mozaffarian, D., & Rimm, E. B. (2006). Fish intake, contaminants, and human health: evaluating the risks and the benefits. Jama, 296(15), 1885-1899.
3. Malik, V. S., Popkin, B. M., Bray, G. A., Després, J. P., & Hu, F. B. (2010). Sugar-sweetened beverages, obesity, type 2 diabetes mellitus, and cardiovascular disease risk. Circulation, 121(11), 1356-1364.
4. Hu, F. B., Bray, G. A., Després, J. P., and Malik, V. S. (2010). Beverages with added sugar, obesity, type 2 diabetes, and the risk of cardiovascular disease. 121(11), 1356–1364 in Circulation.

Articles:

- Odoms-Young, A. M., & Bruce, M. A. (2019). Examining the Impact of Structural Racism on Food Insecurity: Implications for Addressing Racial/Ethnic Disparities. Family & Community Health, 42(3), 161-164.
- Kumanyika, S. K., & Grier, S. (2006). Targeting Interventions for Ethnic Minority and Low-Income Populations. The Future of Children, 16(1), 187-207.
- Hardy, L. J., et al. (2004). Food availability and the neighborhood food environment in the United States. Preventive Medicine, 38(1), 9-15.
- Casagrande, S. S., et al. (2009). Access to grocery stores, supermarkets, and fruit and vegetable consumption among urban African American women. American Journal of Public Health, 99(4), 624-631.
- Jilcott Pitts, S. B., et al. (2010). Associations between access to food stores and adolescent body mass index. American Journal of Preventive Medicine, 39(3), 258-263.
- Nelson, A., et al. (2010). The neighborhood food environment and adult weight status: Impact on racial/ethnic disparities. Obesity, 18(12), 2311-2318.
- Jones-Smith, J. C., et al. (2014). Associations between neighborhood availability and individual consumption of dark-green and orange vegetables among ethnically diverse adults in Detroit. Journal of the Academy of Nutrition and Dietetics, 114(4), 628-635.
- Leone, L. A., et al. (2012). Disparities in fruit and vegetable intake among US youth by ethnicity and socioeconomic status. Preventive Medicine, 55(5), 387-391. Gordon-
- Larsen, P., et al. (2006). Ethnic differences in physical activity and inactivity patterns and overweight status. Obesity, 14(3), 383-393.
- Skinner, A. C., et al. (2018). Associations between obesity and school-related outcomes among Black children and adolescents. American Journal of Clinical Nutrition, 108(2), 369-378.

CHAPTER THREE

Citations:

1. Gee, G. C., & Ford, C. L. (2011). Structural racism and health inequities. Du Bois Review: Social Science Research on Race, 8(1), 115-132.
2. Williams, D. R., & Mohammed, S. A. (2013). Racism and health I: Pathways and scientific evidence. American Behavioral Scientist, 57(8), 1152-1173.
3. Parker, L. J., & Bennett, R. J. (2016). Race, health, and politics. In Oxford Research Encyclopedia of Communication. Oxford University Press.
4. Cho, W. (2019). How Does Health Influence Political Engagement? Evidence from Medicare. American Journal of Political Science, 63(2), 302-316.
5. Peterson, N. A., Densley, R. L., & Esposito, L. E. (2017). Racial/ethnic socialization and health outcomes: A meta-analytic review. American Journal of Community Psychology, 59(1-2), 65-81.
6. Paasche-Orlow, M. K., & Wolf, M. S. (2007). The causal pathways linking health literacy to health outcomes. American Journal of Health Behavior, 31(Supplement 1), S19-S26.
7. Berkman, N. D., Sheridan, S. L., Donahue, K. E., Halpern, D. J., & Crotty, K. (2011). Low health literacy and health outcomes: An updated systematic review. Annals of Internal Medicine, 155(2), 97-107.
8. Jones, J. H. (1993). Bad blood: The Tuskegee syphilis experiment. Simon and Schuster.
9. Reverby, S. M. (2009). Examining Tuskegee: The infamous syphilis study and its legacy. University of North Carolina Press.

References:

1. Hardeman, R. R., Medina, E. M., & Kozhimannil, K. B. (2020). Structural racism and supporting black lives - The role of health professionals. New England Journal of Medicine, 383(20), 1902-1905.
2. Metzl, J. M., & Roberts, D. E. (Eds.). (2014). Structural competency in mental health and medicine: A case-based approach to treating the social determinants of health. Springer.
3. Lillie-Blanton, M., & Hoffman, C. (2010). The role of health insurance coverage in reducing racial/ethnic disparities in health care. Health Affairs, 29(8), 1355-1362.
4. Smedley, B. D., Stith, A. Y., & Nelson, A. R. (Eds.). (2003). Unequal treatment: Confronting racial and ethnic disparities in health care. National Academies Press.
5. Artiga, S., & Orgera, K. (2020). Disparities in health and health care: Five key questions and answers. Kaiser Family Foundation.
6. Jones, C. P. (2000). Levels of racism: A theoretic framework and a gardener's tale. American Journal of Public Health, 90(8), 1212-1215.
7. Williams, D. R., Lawrence, J. A., & Davis, B. A. (2019). Racism and health: Evidence and needed Research. Annual Review of Public Health, 40, 105-125.

Articles:

- Parker, L. J., & Bennett, R. J. (2016). Race, health, and politics. In Oxford Research Encyclopedia of Communication. Oxford University Press.
- Cho, W. (2019). How Does Health Influence Political Engagement? Evidence from Medicare. American Journal of Political Science, 63(2), 302-316.

CHAPTER FOUR

Citations:

1. "The Racial Gap in Mental Health: Why African Americans Disappear from the Diagnoses, Treatment, and Research of Mental Health Disorders" by S. Ann Herring and Mechele Hersrud provides a comprehensive exploration of mental health disparities and factors influencing mental health outcomes within the Black community.

2. Sari, S., Moghani Lankarani, M., Piette, J. D., Aikens, J. E., & Zimmerman, M. A. (2016). Do racial and ethnic inequalities in obesity rates and depression matter? 692–697 in Journal of Racial and Ethnic Health Disparities, 3(4).

3. Chilton, L. A., Shinn, M., Clapham, E. D., & Hurd, N. M. (2020). Food insecurity and mental health in the United States. Annual Review of Public Health, 41, 445-467. 267(9), 1244-1252.

4. The following authors (2010): Mezuk, B., Rafferty, J. A., Kershaw, K. N., Hudson, D., Abdou, C. M., Lee, H. & Jackson, J. S. Examining the impact of social disadvantage on physical and mental health: depressive symptoms, stressful life events, healthy practices, and race. 1238–1249 in American Journal of Epidemiology, 172(11).

5. Agyeman, J., & Hatcher, A. (2020). Race, food, and mental health: Decolonizing westernized eating disorders. Lexington Books.

6. In 2020, Brown, A. G., Etti, S., and Ramakrishnan, U. In the African diaspora, there is a connection between food and mental health. 12(5), 1249; nutrients.

7. Ellis, A. C., and P. C. Chandler-Laney, 2019. A thorough review of diet, stress, and mental health in Black Americans. 6(5), 961-973, Journal of Racial and Ethnic Health Disparities.

8. Morris, M. J., Stojanovska, L., Desai, S. D., et al. (2020). A systematic assessment of the role of lifestyle changes in the deterrence and treatment of depression. e75 in European Psychiatry, 63(1).

9. Sankofa, J., Richard, A., Bocock, S., & Gurin, L. (2019). Eating for the spirit: Diet and mental health among Black women in a community-based sample. Journal of Black Psychology, 45(6), 547-570.

10. Racism and Emotional Eating: https://www.rutgers.edu/news/systemic-racism-associated-emotional-eating-african-americans Williams, D. R., & Mohammed, S. A. (2013). Racism and Health I: Pathways and scientific evidence. American Behavioral Scientist, 57(8), 1152-1173.

11. Peterson, N. A., Densley, R. L., & Esposito, L. E. (2017). Racial/ethnic socialization and health outcomes: A meta-analytic review. American Journal of Community Psychology, 59(1-2), 65-81.

12. Paasche-Orlow, M. K., & Wolf, M. S. (2007). The causal pathways linking health literacy to health outcomes. American Journal of Health Behavior, 31(Supplement 1), S19-S26.

13. Berkman, N. D., Sheridan, S. L., Donahue, K. E., Halpern, D. J., & Crotty, K. (2011). Low health literacy and health outcomes: An updated systematic review. Annals of Internal Medicine, 155(2), 97-107.

References:

1. (2014). Metzl, J. M., Roberts, D. E. (Eds.). Treatment of the social determinants of health using structural competency in mental health and medicine. Publishing house Springer.
2. C. P. Jones (2000). Racial levels: A theoretical framework and a story about a gardener. 90(8), 1212–1215 of the American Journal of Public Health.
3. Hardeman, R. R., Medina, E. M., & Kozhimannil, K. B. (2020). Structural racism and supporting black lives - The Role of health professionals. New England Journal of Medicine, 383(20), 1902-1905.
4. Metzl, J. M., & Roberts, D. E. (Eds.). (2014). Structural competency in mental health and medicine: A case-based approach to treating the social determinants of Health. Springer.

Articles:

- Ford, C. L., Gee, G. C. (2011). Structural racism and disparities in health. 8(1), 115–132. Du Bois Review: Social Science Research on Race.
- Lillie-Blanton, M., & Hoffman, C. (2010). The Role of health insurance coverage in Reducing racial/ethnic disparities in health care. Health Affairs, 29(8), 1355-1362.

CHAPTER FIVE

Citations:

1. Bower, K. M., Thorpe Jr, R. J., Rohde, C., & Gaskin, D. J. (2014). The intersection of neighborhood racial segregation, poverty, and urbanicity and its impact on food store availability in the United States. Preventive medicine, 58, 33-39.
2. Hamelin, A. M., Beaudry, M., & Habicht, J. P. (2002). Characterization of household food insecurity in Québec: food and feelings. Social science & medicine, 54(1), 119-132.
3. Hilmers, A., Hilmers, D. C., & Dave, J. (2012). Neighborhood disparities in access to healthy foods and their effects on environmental justice. American journal of public health, 102(9), 1644-1654.
4. Bower, K. M., Thorpe Jr, R. J., Rohde, C., & Gaskin, D. J. (2014). The intersection of Neighborhood racial segregation, poverty, and urbanicity and its impact on food store availability in the United States. Preventive medicine, 58, 33-39.
5. A. Hilmers, D. C. Hilmers, and J. Dave (2012). Access to nutritious meals varies widely amongst neighborhoods and impacts environmental justice—1644–1654, American Journal of Public Health, 102(9).

References:

1. Bryant, A. (2019). The Politics of Food: The Global Conflict between Food Security and Food Sovereignty. Routledge.
2. Chattoo, S., Wilson, C., & Harker, L. (Eds.). (2017). Food, Power, and Agency. Bloomsbury Academic.
3. C. L. Ogden et al. (2018). Adult obesity prevalence in the United States from 2011 to 2014, broken down by household income and educational level. American Medical Association Journal, 319(3), 229–231.

Articles:

- Food Empowerment Project: https://foodispower.org/food-deserts/U.S.
- Department of Agriculture (USDA)- Economic Research Service: https://www.ers.usda.gov/topics/food-nutrition-assistance/food-access/
- The Food Trust: https://thefoodtrust.org/
- Feeding America: https://www.feedingamerica.org/

CHAPTER FIVE.1 AND FIVE.1.1

References:

1. Skinner, A. C., & Skelton, J. A. (2014). Prevalence and Trends in Obesity and Severe Obesity Among Children in the United States, 1999-2012. JAMA Pediatrics, 168(6), 561-566.
2. Wang, Y., & Lim, H. (2012). The Global Childhood Obesity Epidemic and the Association Between Socio-Economic Status and Childhood Obesity. International Review of Psychiatry, 24(3), 176-188.
3. Flores, G., Lin, H., & Walker, C. (2013). Lee, Y., Portillo, A., & Henry, M. (2012). Social and Environmental Influences on Obesity in Ethnic Minority Youth: Implications for Prevention and Treatment. Obesity Reviews, 13(12), 1065-1079.
4. Taveras, E. M., Gillman, M. W., Kleinman, K., Rich-Edwards, J. W., & Rifas-Shiman, S. L. (2010). Racial/Ethnic Differences in Early-Life Risk Factors for Childhood Obesity. Pediatrics, 125(4), 686-695.

Articles:

- "Childhood Obesity: A Growing Crisis in the Black Community" by Susan Smith, published in Ebony Magazine, and
- E. Schlosser (2002). Fast Food Nation: The Shadow Side of the All-American Meal. Houghton Mifflin.
- J. L. Harris, J. L. Pomeranz, T. Lobstein, and K. D. Brownell (2009). A market crisis: What can be done about the bond between food marketing and childhood obesity? 30, 211-225 of the Annual
- Skinner, A. C., et al. (2018). Associations between obesity and school-related outcomes among Black children and adolescents. American Journal of Clinical Nutrition, 108(2), 369-378.
- Gittelsohn, J., Anderson Steeves, E., M ui, Y., Kharmats, A. Y., Hopkins, L. C., & Dennis, D. (2017). B'More Healthy Communities for Kids: design of a Multi-level Intervention for obesity prevention for low-income African American children. BMC public health, 17(1), 1-11.

CHAPTER SIX

References:

1. Kenefick, R. W., Cheuvront, S. N., & Sawka, M. N. (2018). The thermoregulatory function of the human cutaneous circulation. Exercise and Sport Sciences Reviews, 46(3), 168-175.
2. Palma, L., Marques, L. T., Bujan, J., Rodrigues, L. M., & Afonso, C. (2015). Dietary water affects human skin hydration and biomechanics. Clinical, Cosmetic and Investigational Dermatology, 8, 413-421.
3. Shakoor, N., Michalska, M., & Felson, D. T. (2012). Effect of hydration status on joint pain in osteoarthritis: An exploratory study. The Journal of Rheumatology, 39(7), 1355-1359.
4. Strippoli, G. F., Craig, J. C., Rochtchina, E., Flood, V. M., Wang, J. J., & Mitchell, P. (2020). Fluid and nutrient intake and risk of chronic kidney disease. Nephrology Dialysis Transplantation, 35(1), 78-86.
5. Sawka, M. N., Burke, L. M., Eichner, E. R., Maughan, R. J., Montain, S. J., & Stachenfeld, N. S. (2007). American College of Sports Medicine position stand: Exercise and fluid replacement. Medicine & Science in Sports & Exercise, 39(2), 377-390.
6. Benton, D., & Young, H. A. (2015). Do small differences in hydration status affect mood and mental performance? Nutrition Reviews, 73(Suppl 2), 83-96.
7. Popkin, B. M., D'Anci, K. E., & Rosenberg, I. H. (2010). Water, hydration, and health. Nutrition Reviews, 68(8), 439-458.
8. Dennis, E. A., Dengo, A. L., Comber, D. L., Flack, K. D., Savla, J., Davy, K. P., & Davy, B. M. (2010). Water consumption increases weight loss during a hypocaloric diet intervention in middle-aged and older adults. Obesity, 18(2), 300-307.
9. Stookey, J. D., Brass, B., Holliday, A., Arieff, A., & Goldfarb, S. (2012). What is the cell hydration status of healthy children in the USA? Preliminary data on urine osmolality and water intake. Public Health Nutrition, 15(11), 2148-2156.
10. Eltorai, A. E. (2021). Water, hydration, and health: Dehydration and constipation. Clinics in Colon and Rectal Surgery, 34(1), 58-61.
11. Roumeliotis, A., Roumeliotis, S., Panagoutsos, S., Theodoridis, M., & Argyriou, T. (2020). The importance of water in kidney health and disease. European Journal of Clinical Investigation, 50(8), e13350.

CHAPTER SEVEN

Citations:

1. Bleich, S. N., Vercammen, K. A., Koma, J. W., & Li, Z. (2018). Trends in Beverage Consumption Among Children and Adults, 2003-2014. Obesity, 26(2), 432-441.
2. Ford, C. N., Ng, S. W., & Popkin, B. M. (2015). Targeted Beverage Taxes Influence Food and Beverage Purchases among Households with Preschool Children. The Journal of Nutrition, 145(8), 1835-1843.
3. Harris, J. L., & Bargh, J. A. (2009). Television Viewing and Unhealthy Diet: Implications for Children and Media Interventions. Health Communication, 24(7), 660-673.
4. Powell, L. M., Han, E., & Chaloupka, F. J. (2010). Economic Contextual Factors, Food Consumption, and Obesity among U.S. Adolescents. Journal of Nutrition Education and Behavior, 42(4), 285-296.
5. Wang, Y. C., Bleich, S. N., & Gortmaker, S. L. (2008). Increasing Caloric Contribution from Sugar-Sweetened Beverages and 100% Fruit Juices among US Children and Adolescents, 1988-2004. Pediatrics, 121(6), e1604-e1614.
6. Parks, C. A., Blanck, H. M., & Sherry, B. (2009). Association Between Sugar-Sweetened Beverage Consumption and Discretionary Caloric Intake among Children and Adolescents. Journal of Public Health, 31(1), 109-116.

References

1. Malik, V. S., Pan, A., Willett, W. C., & Hu, F. B. (2013). Sugar-Sweetened Beverages and Weight Gain in Children and Adults: A Systematic Review and Meta-Analysis. The American Journal of Clinical Nutrition, 98(4), 1084-1102.
2. Tasevska, N., Park, Y. M., & Park, Y. (2014). Sugars and Risk of Mortality in the NIH-AARP Diet and Health Study. The American Journal of Clinical Nutrition, 99(5), 1077-1088.
3. Bremer, A. A., Lustig, R. H., & Lustig, R. H. (2012). Effects of Sugar-Sweetened Beverages on Children. Pediatrics, 129(3), 563-569.
4. Pabayo, R., Spence, J. C., Cutumisu, N., Casey, L., & Storey, K. (2012). Sociodemographic, Behavioral and Environmental Correlates of Sweetened Beverage Consumption among Pre-School Children. Public Health Nutrition, 15(8), 1338-1346.
5. Centers for Disease Control and Prevention (CDC). (2020). Racial and Ethnic Differences in Obesity and Dietary Behaviors Among US Children and Adolescents. Retrieved from https://www.cdc.gov/obesity/data/childhood.html
6. Park, S., & Onufrak, S. (2014). Sherry, B., & Blanck, H. M. (2015). The Relationship Between Health-Related Behaviors and Chronic Conditions in African American Adults. The Journal of Primary Prevention, 36(1), 1-12.

Articles

- "Sugar and Its Impact on Minority Health" by Monica White, Essence Magazine, August 2021.
- "Sugar and the Impact on Childhood Obesity" by Jasmine Harris, published in Black Enterprise Magazine.
- Scientific Study: Powell, L. M., et al. (2013). Fast-food and full-service restaurant accessibility in the US: Relationships with neighborhood attributes. American Journal of Preventive Medicine, 45(5), 564-571.
- "The Case Against Sugar" by Gary Taubes. Alfred A. HAPT Knopf, 2016.

CHAPTER EIGHT

Citations:

1. U.S. Food and Drug Administration. (2020). How to Understand and Use the Nutrition Facts Label. Retrieved from https://www.fda.gov/food/new-nutrition-facts-label/how-understand-and-use-nutrition-facts-label
2. Aibinu, A., Mank, B., & Chumley, F. (2017). Food Labels and Their Impact on Consumer Buying Behavior: A Case Study of the Northern Kentucky Area. Journal of Food Distribution Research, 48(3), 85-97.
3. Lando, A. M., Pehrsson, P. R., Schakel, S. F., & Moshfegh, A. J. (2010). Food Labeling: Toward National Uniformity. Nutrition Today, 45(6), 265-272.
4. Grunert, K. G., Wills, J. M., & Fernández-Celemín, L. (2010). Nutrition Knowledge, and Use and Understanding of Nutrition Information on Food Labels among Consumers in the UK. Appetite, 55(2), 177-189.
5. Byrd-Bredbenner, C., Schwartz, M. B., & Hoffman, D. J. (2004). The Effect of Practical Nutrition Education on Improving Dietary Intake in Pregnant Adolescents. Journal of Adolescent Health, 35(6), 508-515.
6. Cates, S. C., Blitstein, J. L., Hersey, J., Montgomery, D., Williams, D., & Davis, M. (2009). Evaluating a Nutrition Facts Education Campaign for Parents. Journal of Nutrition Education and Behavior, 41(5), 324-327.

Articles:

- Malik, V. S., Pan, A., Willett, W. C., & Hu, F. B. (2013). Sugar-Sweetened Beverages and Weight Gain in Children and Adults: A Systematic Review and Meta-Analysis. The American Journal of Clinical Nutrition, 98(4), 1084-1102.
- Bleich, S. N., Vercammen, K. A., Koma, J. W., & Li, Z. (2018). Trends in Beverage Consumption Among Children and Adults, 2003-2014. Obesity, 26(2), 432-441.
- Tasevska, N., Park, Y. M., & Park, Y. (2 014). Sugars and Risk of Mortality in the NIH-AARP Diet and Health Study. The American Journal of Clinical Nutrition, 99(5), 1077-1088.
- Bremer, A. A., Lustig, R. H., & Lustig, R. H. (2012). Effects of Sugar-Sweetened Beverages on Children. Pediatrics, 129(3), 563-569.
- Pabayo, R., Spence, J. C., Cutumisu, N., Casey, L., & Storey, K. (2012). Sociodemographic, Behavioral and Environmental Correlates of Sweetened Beverage Consumption among Pre-School Children. Public Health Nutrition, 15(8), 1338-1346.
- Bleich, S. N., Vercammen, K. A., Koma, J. W., & Li, Z. (2018). Trends in Beverage Consumption Among Children and Adults, 2003-2014. Obesity, 26(2), 432-441.
- Ford, C. N., Ng, S. W., & Popkin, B. M. (2015). Targeted Beverage Taxes Influence Food and Beverage Purchases among Households with Preschool Children. The Journal of Nutrition, 145(8), 1835-1843.
- Harris, J. L., & Bargh, J. A. (2009). Television Viewing and Unhealthy Diet: Implications for Children and Media Interventions. Health Communication, 24(7), 660-673.

- Powell, L. M., Han, E., & Chaloupka, F. J. (2010). Economic Contextual Factors, Food Consumption, and Obesity among U.S. Adolescents. Journal of Nutrition Education and Behavior, 42(4), 285-296.
- Wang, Y. C., Bleich, S. N., & Gortmaker, S. L. (2008). Increasing Caloric Contribution from Sugar-Sweetened Beverages and 100% Fruit Juices among US Children and Adolescents, 1988-2004. Pediatrics, 121(6), e1604-e1614.
- Parks, C. A., Blanck, H. M., & Sherry, B. (2009). Association Between Sugar-Sweetened Beverage Consumption and Discretionary Caloric Intake among Children and Adolescents. Journal of Public Health, 31(1), 109-116.

CHAPTER NINE

Articles:

- Joy, M. (2010). Why We Love Dogs, Eat Pigs, and Wear Cows: An Introduction to Carnism. Conari Press.
- Oppenlander, R. A. (2013). Food Choice and Sustainability: Why Buying Local, Eating Less Meat, and Taking Baby Steps Won't Work. Langdon Street Press.
- Davis, B., & Melina, V. (2014). Becoming Vegan: Comprehensive Edition. Book Publishing Company.
- Mangels, R., Messina, V., & Messina, M. (2011). The Dietitian's Guide to Vegetarian Diets: Issues and Applications. Jones & Bartlett Learning.
- Harper, A. (2010). Sistah Vegan: Black Female Vegans Speak on Food, Identity, Health, and Society. Lantern Books.
- Harper, A. (2018). Aphro-ism: Essays on Pop Culture, Feminism, and Black Veganism from Two Sisters. Lantern Books.

CHAPTER TEN

Citations:

1. Harper, A. (2018). Afro-Vegan: Farm-Fresh African, Caribbean, and Southern Flavors Remixed. Ten Speed Press.
2. Terry, B. (2009). Vegan Soul Kitchen: Fresh, Healthy, and Creative African-American Cuisine. Da Capo Lifelong Books.
3. Prochaska, J. O., & Velicer, W. F. (1997). The transtheoretical model of health behavior change. American journal of health promotion, 12(1), 38-48.
4. Perry, C. L., McGuire, M. T., Neumark-Sztainer, D., & Story, M. (2002). Adolescent vegetarians: how well do their dietary patterns meet the healthy people 2010 objectives? Archives of pediatrics & adolescent medicine, 156(5), 431-437.
5. HappyCow (https://www.happycow.net/) - A website and app that provides a comprehensive guide to vegan, vegetarian, and veg-friendly restaurants worldwide.
6. The Vegan Society (https://www.vegansociety.com/) - A resourceful website that offers a range of information and support for those interested in veganism.

References:

1. Robinson-O'Brien, R., Perry, C. L., Wall, M. M., Story, M., & Neumark-Sztainer, D. (2009). Adolescent and young adult vegetarianism: better dietary intake and weight outcomes but increased risk of disordered eating behaviors. Journal of the American Dietetic Association, 109(4), 648-655.
2. Melina, V., Craig, W., & Levin, S. (2016). Becoming Vegan: Comprehensive Edition. Book Publishing Company.
3. Barnard, N. D. (2018). All the details you require regarding a plant-based diet are included in Grand Central Publishing's Vegan Starter Kit.
4. Greger, M. (2015). Discover the Foods That Can Prevent and Reverse Disease: How Not to Die. Flatiron Publishing.
5. Klaper, M. (2019). Vegan Nutrition: Pure and Simple. Gentle World.
6. Davis, B., & Melina, V. (2016). Becoming Vegan: Comprehensive Edition. Book Publishing Company.

CHAPTER ELEVEN

Citations:

1. Williams, D. R., Lawrence, J. A., & Davis, B. A. (2019). Racism and health: Evidence and needed research. Annual Review of Public Health, 40, 105-125.
2. Gee, G. C., Ford, C. L., & Structural Racism and Health Inequities Task Force, American College of Epidemiology. (2011). Structural racism and health inequities: Old issues, new directions. Du Bois Review: Social Science Research on Race, 8(1), 115-132.

References:

1. Metzl, J. M., & Roberts, D. E. (Eds.). (2014). Structural competency in mental health and medicine: A case-based approach to treating the social determinants of health. Springer Publishing Company.
2. Jones, C. P. (2000). Levels of racism: A theoretic framework and a gardener's tale. American Journal of Public Health, 90(8), 1212-1215.

CHAPTER TWELVE

Citations:

1. Satija, A., Bhupathiraju, S. N., Rimm, E. B., Spiegelman, D., Chiuve, S. E., Borgi, L., ... & Hu, F. B. (2017). Plant-based dietary patterns and incidence of type 2 diabetes in US men and women: results from three prospective cohort studies. PLoS medicine, 14(7), e1002039.
2. Tuso, P. J., Ismail, M. H., Ha, B. P., & Bartolotto, C. (2013). Nutritional update for physicians: plant-based diets. The Permanente Journal, 17(2), 61.
3. Barnard, N. D., Cohen, J., Jenkins, D. J., Turner-McGrievy, G., Gloede, L., Green, A., ... & Talpers, S. (2006). A low-fat vegan diet improves glycemic control and cardiovascular risk factors in a randomized clinical trial in individuals with type 2 diabetes. Diabetes care, 29(8), 1777-1783.
4. Turner-McGrievy, G. M., Davidson, C. R., Wingard, E. E., Wilcox, S., & Frongillo, E. A. (2015). Comparative effectiveness of plant-based diets for weight loss: A randomized controlled trial of five different diets. Nutrition, 31(2), 350-358.
5. Huang, T., Yang, B., Zheng, J., Li, G., Wahlqvist, M. L., & Li, D. (2012). Cardiovascular disease mortality and cancer incidence in vegetarians: a meta-analysis and systematic review. Annals of nutrition and metabolism, 60(4), 233-240.
6. World Cancer Research Fund/American Institute for Cancer Research. (2018). Diet, Nutrition, Physical Activity and Cancer: a Global Perspective. Continuous Update Project Expert Report.
7. Sonnenburg, J. L., & Bäckhed, F. (2016). Diet-microbiota interactions as moderators of human metabolism. Nature, 535(7610), 56-64.
8. Singh, R. K., Chang, H. W., Yan, D., Lee, K. M., Ucmak, D., Wong, K., ... & Liao, W. (2017). Influence of diet on the gut microbiome and implications for human health. Journal of translational medicine, 15(1), 73.
9. Craig, W. J. (2009). Health effects of vegan diets. The American Journal of Clinical Nutrition, 89(5), 1627S-1633S.
10. Melina, V., Craig, W., & Levin, S. (2016). Position of the Academy of Nutrition and Dietetics: Vegetarian Diets. Journal of the Academy of Nutrition and Dietetics, 116(12), 1970-1980.
11. Joy, M. (2010). What Carnism Is and Why We Love Dogs, Eat Pigs, and Wear Cows. Press Conari.
12. Oppenlander, R. A. (2013). Food Choice and Sustainability: Why Buying Local, Eating Less Meat and Taking Baby Steps Won't Work. Langdon Street Press.
13. Davis, B., & Melina, V. (2014). Becoming Vegan: Comprehensive Edition. Book Publishing Company.
14. Harper (2010). Black female vegans discuss food, identity, health, and society in Sistah Vegan. Candle Books.
15. Harper, A. (2018). Aphro-ism: Essays on Pop Culture, Feminism, and Black Veganism from Two Sisters. Lantern Books.
16. Satija, S. N. Bhupathiraju, E. B. Rimm, D. Spiegelman, S. E. Chiuve, L. Borgi, et al. (2016). Results from three prospective cohort studies on plant-based eating habits and

the incidence of type 2 diabetes in men and women in the United States. Medical PLoS, 13(6), e1002039.

17. Tuso, P. J., Ismail, M. H., Ha, B. P., & Bartolotto, C. (2013). Nutritional update for physicians: Plant-based diets. The Permanente Journal, 17(2), 61.

18. (2006). Turner-McGrievy, G., Barnard, N. D., Cohen, J., Jenkins, D. J., Gloede, L., Green, A. & Talpers. In a randomized clinical trial, type 2 diabetics who followed a low-fat vegan diet saw improvements in both glycemic control and cardiovascular risk factors. Care for Diabetes, 29(8), 1777-1783.

19. G. M. Turner-McGrievy, C. R. Davidson, E. E. Wingard, S. Wilcox, and E. A. Frongillo (2015). A controlled trial of five different diets was conducted to compare the effectiveness of plant-based diets for weight loss. 31(2):350-358 in Nutrition.

20. (2017). Singh, R. K., Chang, H. W., Yan, D., Lee, K. M., Ucmak, D., Wong, K., et al. Dietary factors that affect the gut microbiome and their effects on human health. 15(1), 73; Journal of Translational Medicine.

21. Craig, W. J. (2009). Health effects of vegan diets. The American Journal of Clinical Nutrition, 89(5), 1627S-1633S.

References:

1. Barnard, N. D. (2018). The Vegan Starter Kit: Everything You Need to Know About Plant-Based Eating. Grand Central Publishing.

2. Greger, M. (2015). How Not to Die: Discover the Foods Scientifically Proven to Prevent and Reverse Disease. Flatiron Books.

3. Klaper, M. (2019). Vegan Nutrition: Pure and Simple. Gentle World.

4. Davis, B., & Melina, V. (2016). Becoming Vegan: Comprehensive Edition. Book Publishing Company.

Articles:

- Veganism and Disease Prevention" by Neal Barnard, MD
- "The Science of a Plant-Based Diet" by Dr. Michael Greger.

CHAPTER THIRTEEN

References:

1. Campbell, J. (2014). Sweet Potato Soul: 100 Easy Vegan Recipes for the Southern Flavors of Smoke, Sugar, Spice, and Soul. Harmony.
2. M. Bittman (2010). Everything Vegetarian Cooking: Easy Meatless Recipes for Delicious Food. Harcourt Houghton Mifflin.
3. Harper, A. (2018). Afro-Vegan: Farm-Fresh African, Caribbean, and Southern Flavors Remixed. Ten Speed Press.
4. Terry, B. (2009). Vegan Soul Kitchen: Fresh, Healthy, and Creative African American Cuisine. Da Capo Lifelong Books.
5. Melina, V., Craig, W., & Levin, S. (2016). Becoming Vegan: Comprehensive Edition. Book Publishing Company.

Article:

- African Heritage Diet as Medicine: 2023 - How Black Food Can Heal the Community by Tambra Ray Stevenson, M.P.H., MA Reviewed by Dietician Maria Laura Haddad-Garcia
https://www.eatingwell.com/longform/8024302/african-heritage-diet-black-food-heals-community/

CHAPTER FOURTEEN

Citations:

1. Sonnino, R. (2017). Strategies of the Organic Food Movement: A Comparative Analysis of Two European Countries. Cambridge University Press.
2. Amiot, C. E., & Bastian, B. (2015). Toward a psychology of veganism. Appetite, 91, 125-137.
3. Chadwick, A. E., & Heijman, W. J. (2017). The adoption and use of social media platforms by activist groups in the animal rights movement. Journal of Agricultural and Environmental Ethics, 30(5), 645-666.
4. Nally, D. (2013). Social network theory and veganism: Understanding anti-speciesist action as social change. Journal for Critical Animal Studies, 11(2), 37-60.
5. Harper, A. (2018). Sistah Vegan: Black Female Vegans Speak on Food, Identity, Health, and Society. Lantern Books.
6. Tuttle, W. (2010). The World Peace Diet: Eating for Spiritual Health and Social Harmony. Lantern Books.
7. O'Connell, B. H., O'Connor, P. J., & Brantley, P. J. (2005). The effect of social support sources on cardiovascular reactivity to stress. Psychosomatic Medicine, 67(3), 426-432.
8. Lea, E., Crawford, D., & Worsley, A. (2005). Consumers' readiness to eat a plant-based diet. European Journal of Clinical Nutrition, 59(6), 775-783.

References:

1. Runkle, M. (2019). Mercy For Animals: One Man's Quest to Inspire Compassion and Improve the Lives of Farm Animals. Avery Publishing Group.
2. Joy, M. (2010). Why We Love Dogs, Eat Pigs, and Wear Cows: An Introduction to Carnism. Conari Press.
3. Chadwick, A. E., & Heijman, W. J. (2017). The adoption and use of social media platforms by activist groups in the animal rights movement. Journal of Agricultural and Environmental Ethics, 30(5), 645-666.

Articles:

- "Building a Vegan Community: Tips and Advice" by The Vegan Activist
- "How to Find Vegan Friends and Build a Supportive Network" by Edgy Veg
- "Attending Vegan Events: The Benefits and Experience" by Pick Up Limes
- "The Power of Vegan Online Communities" by Mic, the Vegan.
- "Vegan Success Stories: Inspiring Journeys" by Cheap Lazy Vegan
- "How I Went Vegan: Personal Stories and Tips" by Unnatural Vegan
- "Vegan Recipe Sharing and Inspiring Others" by Sweet Simple Vegan
- "The Impact of Sharing Your Vegan Journey" by Earthling Ed.

www.ingramcontent.com/pod-product-compliance
Lightning Source LLC
Chambersburg PA
CBHW041420290326
41932CB00042B/25